Med *in* 28

 Your *Practical Guide*
to Mediterranean Cooking

28 DAY MEAL PLAN
100 RECIPES

ALEX JOHNSON

Important Note

The information in this book reflects the author's research, experiences and opinions and is not intended as medical advice. Before beginning any nutritional or exercise program, consult your doctor or physician to ensure it's appropriate for you.

Table *of* Contents

Dinner 91

Vegetarian 93

Poultry 143

Meat 171

Fish 197

Snacks & Sides 225

28 Day Plan 241

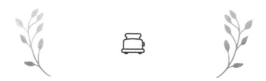

Intro

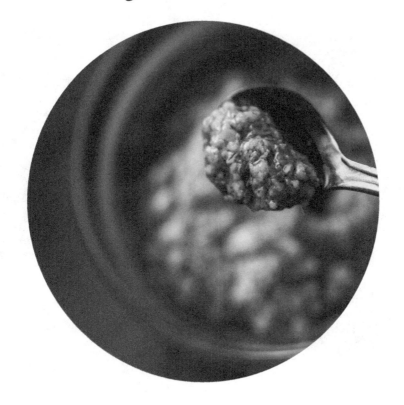

Why Choose the Mediterranean Diet?

When most people think about the word 'diet', they think deprivation. These characteristics don't need to apply to the Mediterranean diet.

Numerous studies show a traditional Mediterranean diet may benefit the conditions such as type 2 diabetes, high blood pressure, raised cholesterol, heart disease and obesity. The Mediterranean diet is one of the easiest diets to adhere to long-term. Drawing from a range of cooking influences, it's delicious flavors and low cost make it a practical solution for most people.

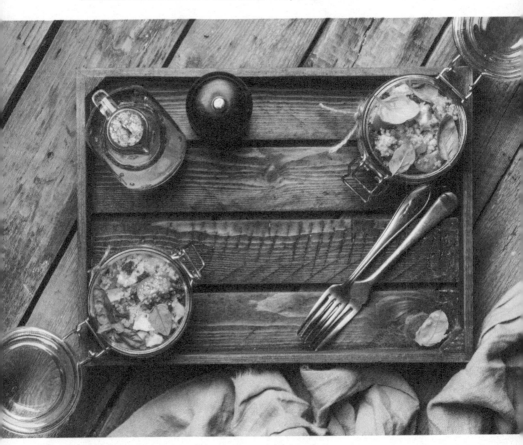

What is the Mediterranean Diet?

The Mediterranean diet represents the dietary pattern usually consumed among the populations bordering the Mediterranean Sea in the early 1960s. These include countries such as Spain, France, Southern Italy, Morocco, Malta, Turkey, Greece and Israel. This means there isn't one single, definitive Mediterranean diet. The Mediterranean diet brings together what each cuisine has in common rather than the differences. The Mediterranean diet is traditionally characterized by:-

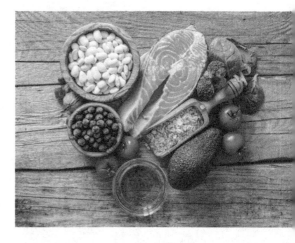

- High monounsaturated to saturated fat ratio, due partly to the high usage of olive oil as the main cooking ingredient.

- High consumption of fruits, vegetables, legumes, nuts and unrefined grains.

- Increased consumption of fish.

- Moderate consumption of dairy (mostly cheese and yogurt).

- Low intake of red wine, primarily during meals (optional).

- Drinking water as your main non-alcoholic beverage.

- Limited intake of red meat and processed foods.

- Snacks made up of fruit, vegetables and unsalted nuts.

- Regular physical activity.

- Sharing meals with other people and enjoying life.

An easy way to understand the proportions of food group servings that make up the Mediterranean diet is through the Mediterranean pyramid.

Overview of The Mediterranean Diet Pyramid

The Mediterranean Diet Pyramid was developed by Oldways, the Harvard School of Public Health, and the World Health Organisation in 1993. It serves as a summary of the eating patterns within the Mediterranean diet and the types and frequency of particular food groups. The pyramid was established after the results of the Seven Countries Study, which was started by American psychologist Ancel Keys in the late 1950s.

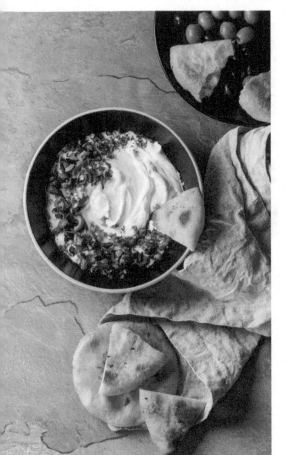

It aimed to study questions about heart and vascular diseases among countries with various traditional eating patterns and lifestyles. The study showed that the dietary patterns in the Mediterranean in the 1960s were associated with low rates of coronary heart disease.

The studies of the elderly showed that a healthy diet and lifestyle, including adequate physical activity, non-smoking and some alcohol consumption was also associated with a low risk of cardiovascular disease.

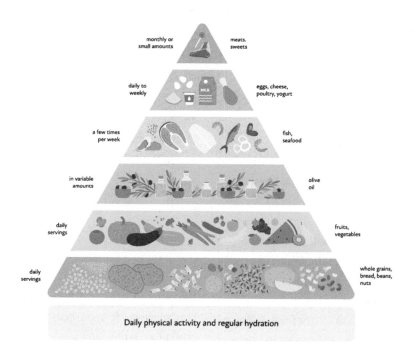

monthly or
small amounts — meats.
sweets

daily to
weekly — eggs, cheese,
poultry, yogurt

a few times
per week — fish,
seafood

in variable
amounts — olive
oil

daily
servings — fruits,
vegetables

daily
servings — whole grains,
bread, beans,
nuts

Daily physical activity and regular hydration

VEGETABLES & FRUITS

Fruit and vegetables are high in vitamins, minerals and fibre. Although the World Health Organization recommends eating at least 5 portions of fruit and vegetables a day, traditionally Greek residents ate on average nine servings. Tinned, dried and frozen fruit or vegetables can all play an important part in the diet. They are high in fiber, antioxidants and vitamins.

CEREALS & GRAINS

Cereals and grains should be whole grain. Examples are wheat, barley, oats, millet, corn and rice. This includes foods such as wholemeal bread, brown rice or pasta. Grains are made up of a germ, endosperm and bran. These are important sources of fiber, potassium and magnesium. Refining grains removes the germ and bran and a lot of the vitamins, minerals and fiber contained within wholegrains.

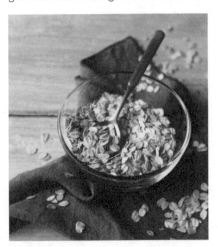

FISH

Oily fish should be eaten at least twice a week. They are high in many nutrients that most people aren't getting enough of, including vitamin A, D and Omega-3 fatty acids, which are found in oily fish.

Omega-3 fatty acids may reduce the risk of heart disease, some cancers and dementia. They are also thought to be helpful for brain development and in the treatment of depression.

White fish is also a good source of protein and is low in saturated fats.

LEGUMES

Legumes are a type of vegetable that grows from a pod. Well-known legumes include peas, beans, chickpeas, lentils and peanuts. They form quite an important part of the Mediterranean Diet and are a useful base for soups and stews. They provide protein, carbohydrates, fiber and vitamins. They are associated with a reduced risk of heart disease.

FATS AND OILS

The Mediterranean diet features olive oil as the primary source of fat. Olive oil provides monounsaturated fat — a type of fat that can help reduce LDL cholesterol levels when used in place of saturated or trans fats.

"Extra-virgin" olive oils — the least processed forms — also contain the highest levels of protective plant compounds that provide antioxidant effects.

The focus of the Mediterranean diet isn't on limiting total fat consumption but rather to make wise choices about the types of fat you eat. The Mediterranean diet discourages saturated fats and trans fats, both of which have been linked to heart disease.

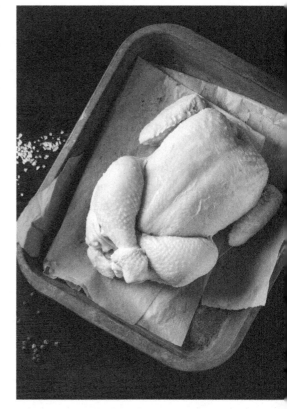

raise blood pressure.

NUTS AND SEEDS

Nuts such as almonds, walnuts and cashews and also seeds such as pumpkin, sunflower and sesame, provide protein, fiber, vitamins and minerals. Nuts are high in fat (approximately 80 percent of their calories come from fat), but most of the fat is unsaturated fat. Because nuts are high in calories, they should not be eaten in large amounts if you're looking to lose weight. Generally a handful a day should suffice. Avoid salted nuts, as salt can

POULTRY

Chicken, turkey and other poultry are high in protein, vitamins and minerals. It is best to remove the skin and visible fat. When white meat is served in processed foods like pies, burgers and fried chicken it is usually higher in animal fat and is not a healthy choice. A chicken's nutrient profile is often affected by its diet. Pasture-raised chickens have higher antioxidant and omega-3 levels, so buy organic and free-range where budget permits.

WINE

The Mediterranean diet traditionally allows moderate amounts of red wine. Current health guidelines for men and women recommend no more than two small glasses of wine daily, preferably with a couple of alcohol-free days during the week. Although red wine has been linked to some health benefits as it contains antioxidants and anti-inflammatory chemicals, none of them are worthy of encouraging alcohol consumption. Red wine contains twice the amount of calories as beer and sugary soft drinks. Excessive consumption may therefore contribute to high-calorie intake and make you gain weight.

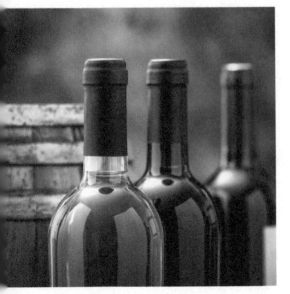

DAIRY

Dairy products are an important

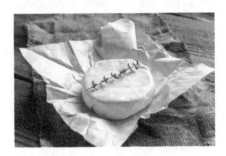

part of the Mediterranean diet. They are listed higher up on the Mediterranean pyramid but are not to be consumed in the same amounts as the whole grain, vegetable, fruit and nut categories. Dairy products contain protein, vitamins A and B12 and calcium. However, some are also high in saturated fat. Choosing lower-fat cheeses such as feta rather than cream cheese or cheddar will reduce your saturated fat intake. Choosing semi-skimmed or skimmed milk rather than full-cream milk is also a lower fat option, but check that extra sugar has not been added to compensate. Greek yogurt is different from regular yogurt in that it is extensively strained to remove the liquid lactose sugar and whey. Greek yogurt can also contain double the protein of regular yogurt while cutting sugar content in half.

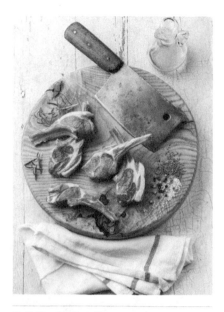

RED MEAT

Red meat such as beef, pork or lamb is eaten in smaller quantities in the Mediterranean Diet than in typical Western diets. Meat does contain high amounts of protein, vitamins and minerals (especially iron) but tends to be higher in fat (particularly saturated fat) compared with poultry. When found in processed foods such as pies and sausages, it is likely to be higher in fat and lower in nutritional value. There is no need to eliminate red meat completely and it can form part of a healthy diet. However, try to keep it as a treat and limit to one meal per week, such as part of a roast dinner, or to make it into a stew or casserole with lots of vegetables. In this way, you are consuming less red meat overall.

SWEETS AND DESSERTS

The Mediterranean diet doesn't deprive you of sweets and desserts. However, try to keep portion sizes small and savor the taste instead, keeping them for occasional treats. Don't gorge! Most sweets and desserts contain lots of sugar — a major contributor to type 2 diabetes and tooth decay. They often contain high levels of saturated fat as well. Although many supermarket desserts contain fruit, they rarely contain enough fruit to count as a portion.

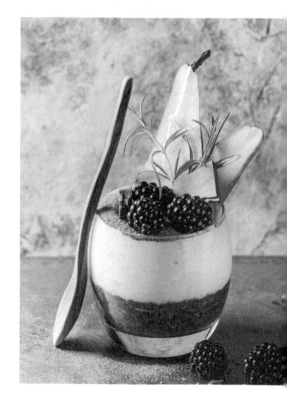

Daily Exercise

Regular exercise strengthens the cardiovascular system, builds muscle and burns extra calories. As a general goal, aim for at least 30 minutes of moderate physical activity most days of the week (5+ times/week). This can include activities such as brisk walking, swimming, mowing the lawn etc or 75+ minutes (2-3 times/week) of vigorous aerobic activity.

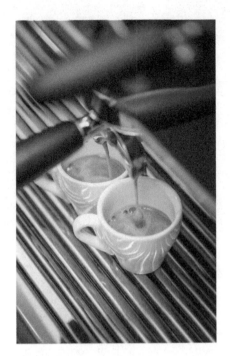

Drinks

Water should be your go-to beverage on a Mediterranean diet. Coffee and tea are also completely acceptable (avoid adding too much extra sugar) and avoid sugar-sweetened beverages and fruit juices, which can be very high in sugar.

The Mediterranean diet traditionally allows moderate amounts of red wine. However, despite red wine consumption being linked with some health benefits, none of them are worthy of encouraging alcohol consumption. There are many other effective ways to improve your health that don't require you to consume something that can be harmful.

Foods to Avoid

- Refined grains: White bread, pasta made with refined wheat, etc.

- Trans fats: Found in margarine and various processed foods.

- Refined oils: Soybean oil, canola oil, cottonseed oil and others.

- Processed meat: Processed sausages, hot dogs etc.

- Added sugar.

No diet no matter how healthy, is not sustainable unless the food is satisfying and exciting. The Mediterranean diet ticks all the boxes. By drawing influences from a number of countries, there are various tastes to experiment with. The recipes are also accessible, using ingredients you can find in your local supermarket.

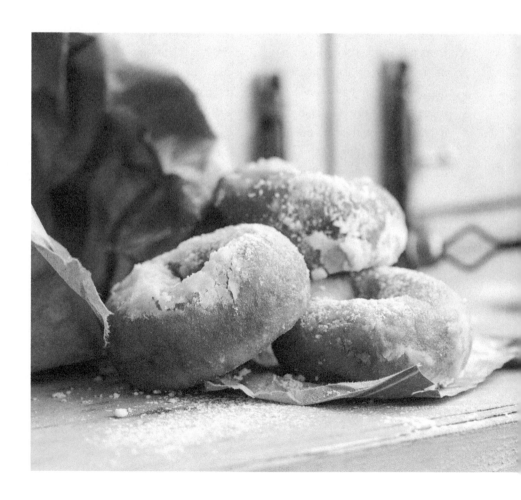

Why You Should Choose Extra Virgin Olive Oil

———

Olive oil is made simply by pressing olives and extracting the oil.

Olive oil contains high amounts of monosaturated fatty acids. When these fats replace saturated and trans fats in your diet, they can help reduce your risk of heart disease. Olive oil has been shown to lower blood pressure and reduce inflammation, with some preliminary evidence suggesting it can help fight cancer and Alzheimer's disease.

However, there are many varieties of olive oil that can cause confusion. Extra virgin olive oil is unrefined and is the highest quality of olive oil. It must be produced via mechanical means without chemical treatment, pass various sensory standards and contain less than 1% of oleic acid.

Most of the olive oils you see on the supermarket shelves containinh 'refined' oil are labelled as 'pure', 'light' or just plain olive oil. The refining process prolongs the shelf life but removes a lot of the goodness from the oil. They are extracted with solvents, treated with heat or even diluted with cheaper oils.

Extra virgin olive oils can be distinguished from refined oils via their fruity and slightly bitter taste.

———

———

Losing Weight with the Mediterranean Diet

A diet is only useful if you're able to stick with it long-term. It should provide lots of choice, restrict certain foods only where necessary and use ingredients that can be sourced from your usual shopping trip.

The problem with many 'fad' diets is that they are unsuitable for long-term use. Most are focused on depriving you in some way. Whether that's cutting carbs, fats, calories or whole food groups, they are often designed to be sustained for only a short time. Although most diets help you shed pounds, many people find they slowly regain the weight they lost and often more than they originally started with.

Common diet approaches include low fat and low carbohydrate.

Low-fat diets have been around for a while. However, healthy fats such as those found in foods like olive oil, nuts and seeds have been found to improve weight loss. Foods rich in good fats help you feel full and they won't trigger the insulin high and crash that most processed carbs do.

Low carbohydrate diets also have problems. Limiting carbs in favor of protein and fat prevents the insulin surge, helping you feel full for longer. However, carb-rich fruits, vegetables and whole grains have been shown to lower the risk of heart disease and even obesity due to their satiety, which is a measure of how well foods fill you up. Diets low in carbohydrates also tend to be high in saturated fat because of the high consumption of red meat.

The Mediterranean diet has a moderate amount of fat, but most of it comes from healthy fats. The carbohydrates in Mediterranean-style diets tend to come from unrefined sources like whole wheat and beans. High consumption of vegetables, fruits, nuts and fish is linked to various health benefits and long-term weight loss. The Mediterranean diet is a good choice if you're looking to keep the weight off whilst developing eating habits scientifically proven to help with heart disease and other health markers.

Tips for Following the Plan

————

Make sure you buy extra virgin olive oil for all of your cooking — it is high in healthy, monounsaturated fats and contains high levels of antioxidants. Anything else, such as 'pure', 'light' or just plain olive oil, is chemically refined to varying degrees and should be avoided.

There are a variety of snack recipes within this book if you want to get creative and treat yourself occasionally, but the cheapest and healthiest option is to stick with fresh fruit and nuts. Nuts particularly can have positive effects on cholesterol due in part to their high content of monounosaturated and polyunsaturated fatty acids. Numerous studies showing how almonds and hazelnuts appear to reduce LDL (bad) cholesterol whilst increasing HDL ("good") cholesterol levels. A small handful a day is absolutely fine. Don't eat too many as they are quite calorie-dense.

You'll notice that the lunch on Sunday is left as 'filler'. This gives some flexibility on weekends in case you're eating out and can't follow an exact meal plan. This will prevent you from buying ingredients you don't end up using.

CLEARING YOUR CUPBOARD

We recommend removing as much processed food, white bread and sweets as possible. If you only have good food in your home, you will only eat good food.

If other family members want to keep these foods around, at least keep them hidden, rather than on worktops.

The saying "out of sight, out of mind" definitely applies here. Having food on display in various areas of the house has been linked to obesity and increased consumption of unhealthy foods.

TRACKING PROGRESS ON THE PLAN?

If you're looking to track weight throughout your diet plan, you should use both progress pictures and weight measurements to track your progress over the course of the 4 weeks.

Although tracking your weight is important, you should focus your attention on the changes within your photos as well. This is because some changes may not be visible on the scales, but may be more visible in the mirror.

Bodyweight tends to fluctuate by a few pounds because of water retention.

This can be affected by hormones as well as the food you eat. It is also possible to gain muscle at the same time as you lose weight, which is particularly common if you recently start exercising or weight training.

This is good! What you really want is to lose body fat, not weight.

Without records of your progress, it can be easy to lose motivation.

Take photos or weigh yourself in similar situations each time, preferably first thing in the morning. This ensures your results aren't influenced by other factors, such as whether or not you have eaten.

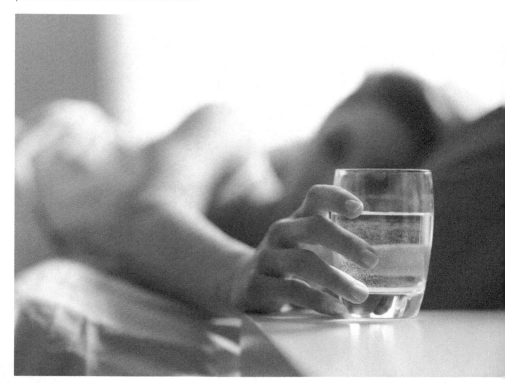

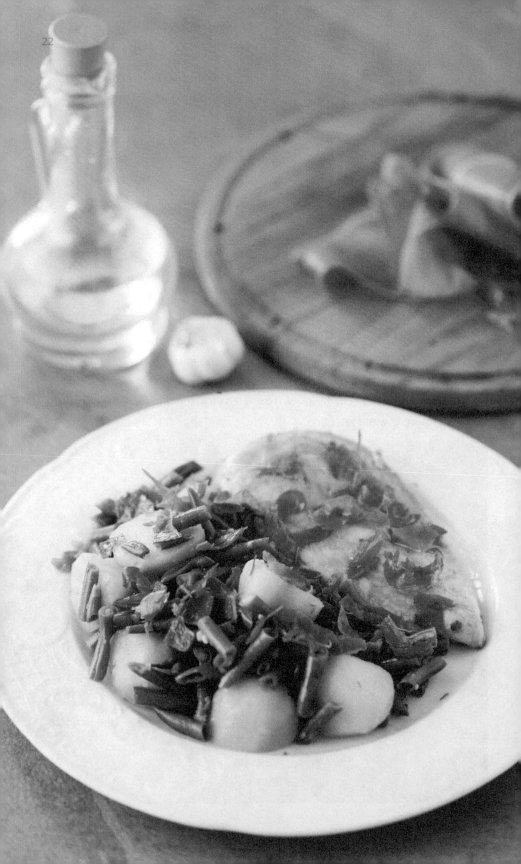

Recipes

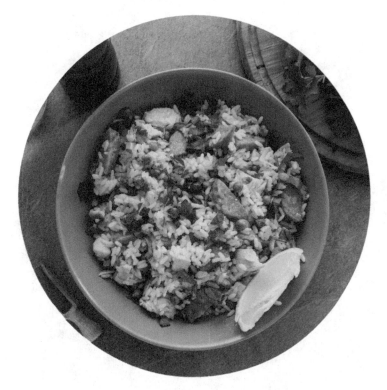

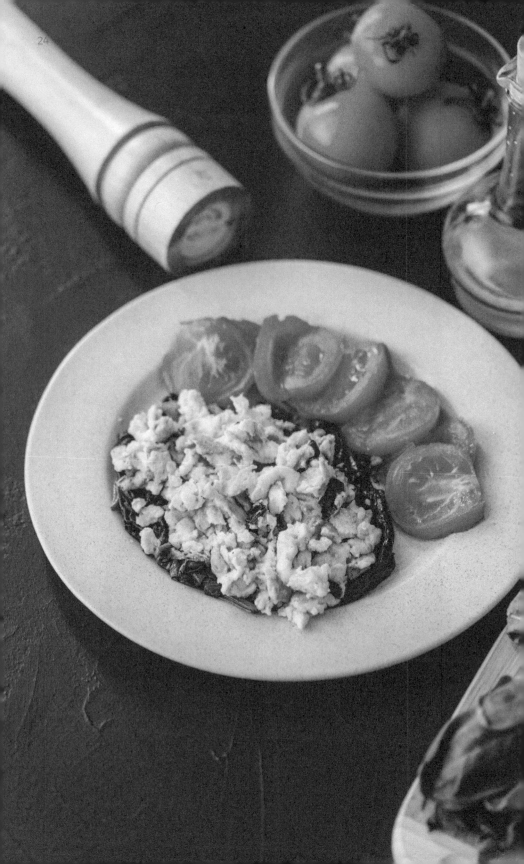

Breakfast

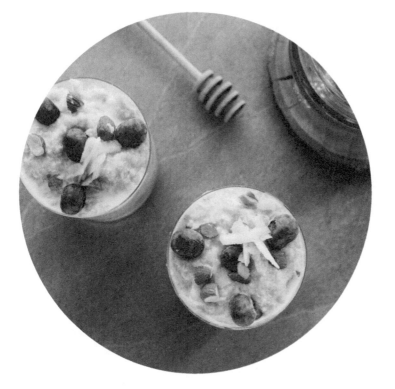

Breakfast Blues Porridge

SUITABLE

Vegetarian

PREP TIME

5 mins

COOK TIME

No Cook

SERVES

2

Nutrition (per serving)	Kcal	Fat	Sat Fat	Carb	Sugar	Fibre	Protein	Salt
	347	15g	3g	42g	14g	10g	15g	0.2g

INGREDIENTS

½ cup / 50g porridge oats

⅚ cup / 200ml milk

½ tsp vanilla extract

2 tbsp Greek yogurt

⅛ cup / 25g chia seeds

¾ cup / 150g blueberries

¼ cup / 25g almonds, flaked

METHOD

01/ Mix the porridge oats, milk, vanilla extract, Greek yogurt and chia seeds in a bowl and soak for one minute. Once the oats have softened, add some of the blueberries.

02/ Place the mixture into two bowls and add any remaining berries and almonds.

Notes:

You can replace the blueberries with other berries.

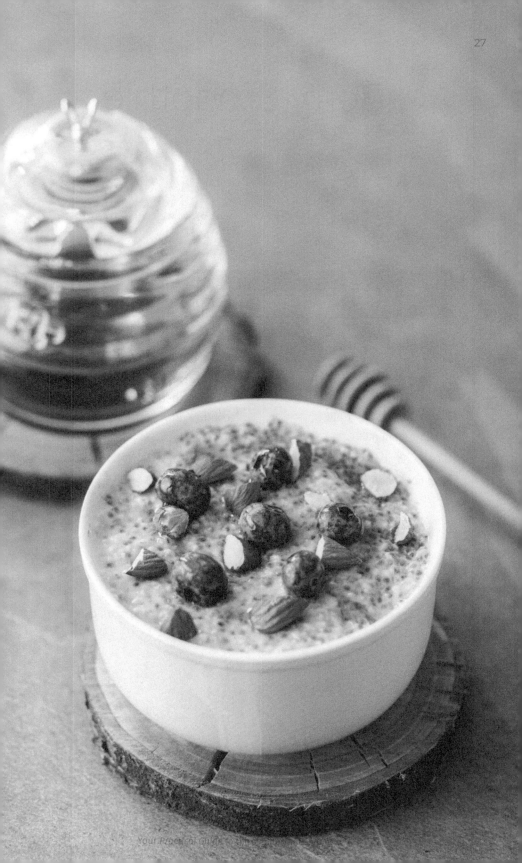

Berry Smoothie

SUITABLE
Vegetarian

PREP TIME
10 mins

COOK TIME
No Cook

SERVES
2

Nutrition (per serving)	Kcal	Fat	Sat Fat	Carb	Sugar	Fibre	Protein	Salt
	207	4g	2g	27g	15g	5g	15g	0.1g

INGREDIENTS

1 ¼ cups / 250g frozen berries

1 cup / 250g Greek yogurt

⅕ cup / 50ml milk

⅕ cup / 15g porridge oats

2 tsp honey *(optional)*

METHOD

01/ Whizz berries, yogurt and milk together until smooth. Stir through porridge oats and pour into glasses. Serve with a drizzle of honey.

Notes:

Try experimenting with different fruits. If too thick, add extra milk.

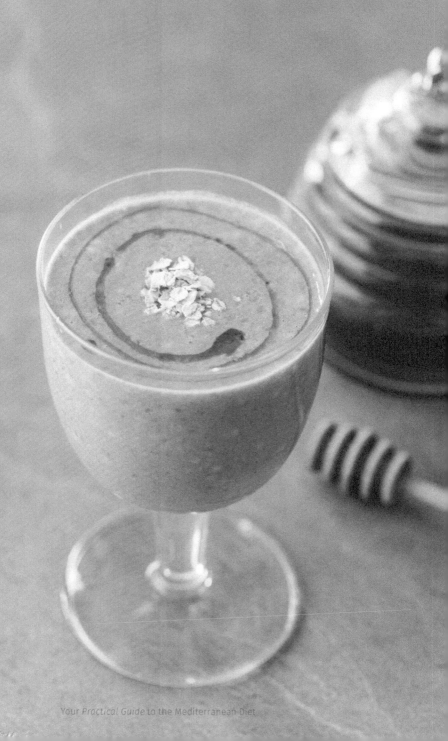

Tomato & Feta Omelette

SUITABLE
Vegetarian

PREP TIME
5 mins

COOK TIME
5 mins

SERVES
2

Nutrition (per serving)	Kcal	Fat	Sat Fat	Carb	Sugar	Fibre	Protein	Salt
	320	20g	7g	21g	15g	6g	19g	1.1g

INGREDIENTS

2 tsp olive oil

4 eggs, beaten

½ cup / 8 cherry tomatoes, chopped

⅓ cup / 50g feta cheese, crumbled

mixed salad leaves, to serve (optional)

METHOD

01/ Heat the oil in a frying pan, add the eggs and cook, swirling them occasionally. After a few minutes, scatter the feta and tomatoes. Cook for another minute before serving.

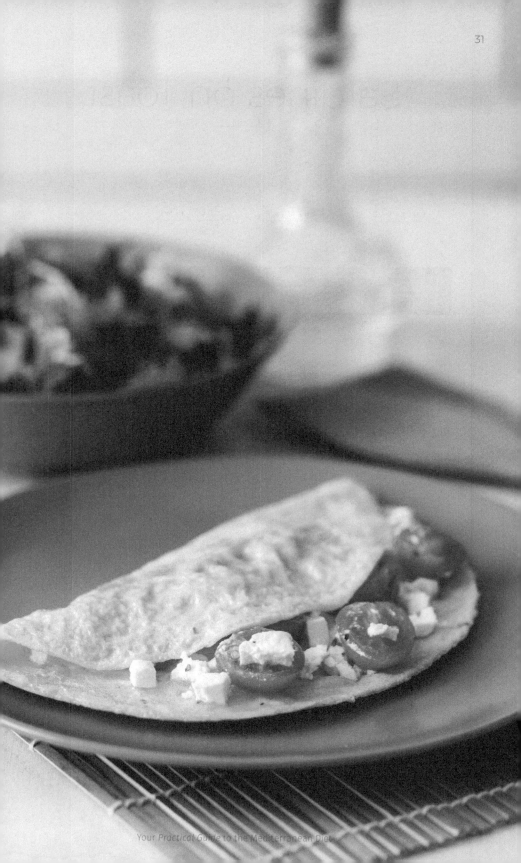

Sardines on Toast

SUITABLE

Quick

PREP TIME

5 mins

COOK TIME

5 mins

SERVES

2

Nutrition (per serving)	Kcal	Fat	Sat Fat	Carb	Sugar	Fibre	Protein	Salt
	480	19g	3g	46g	6g	7g	32g	2.0g

INGREDIENTS

1 tbsp olive oil

1 onion

1 garlic clove, crushed

1 red chilli, chopped and deseeded

1 lemon, juice and zest

2 x 120g / 4 oz cans of sardines in olive oil

4 slices of brown bread

small bunch of parsley, chopped

METHOD

01/ Heat the oil in a frying pan, cook onions for a few minutes before adding the garlic, red chilli and lemon zest.

02/ Add sardines and heat for a few minutes until warm.

03/ Toast the bread. Add parsley and a squeeze of lemon juice to the sardines. Divide between toast before serving.

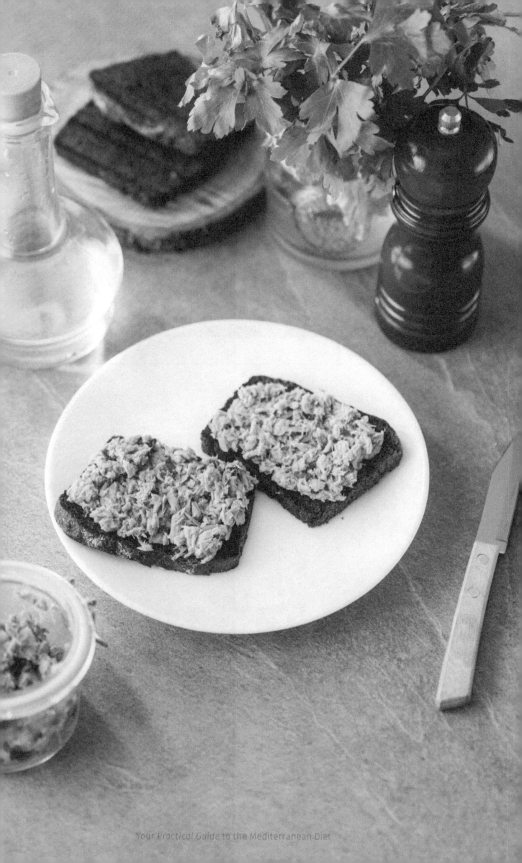

Zucchini, Feta & Mint Salad

SUITABLE
Vegetarian

PREP TIME
10 mins

COOK TIME
No Cook

SERVES
2

Nutrition (per serving)	Kcal	Fat	Sat Fat	Carb	Sugar	Fibre	Protein	Salt
	210	20g	6g	6g	3g	2g	6g	0.7g

INGREDIENTS

1 zucchini / courgette

½ cup / 50g rocket / arugula leaves

⅓ cup / 50g feta cheese, crumbled

bunch of mint, leaves picked

2 tbsp olive oil

METHOD

01/ Peel the zucchini into ribbons with a potato peeler. Add arugula leaves, mint and feta and drizzle with olive oil.

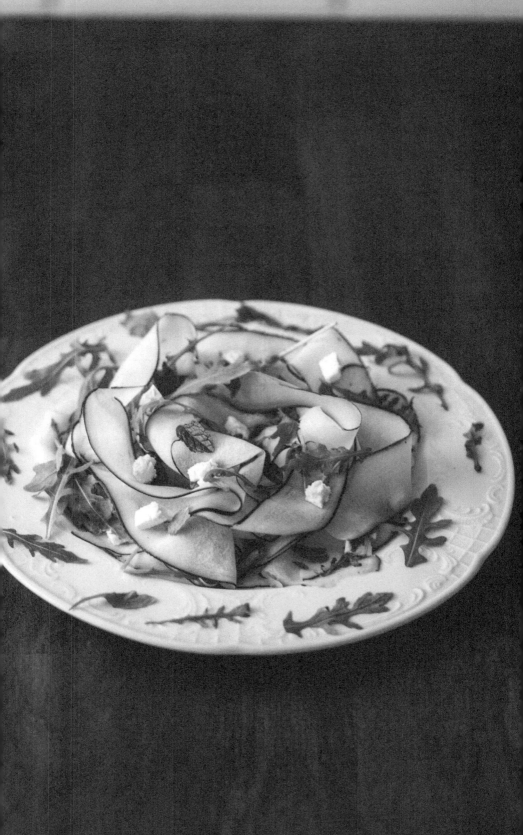

Apple & Blueberry Bircher Pots

SUITABLE
Vegetarian

PREP TIME
5 mins

COOK TIME
No Cook

SERVES
2

Nutrition (per serving)	Kcal	Fat	Sat Fat	Carb	Sugar	Fibre	Protein	Salt
	199	2g	0.5g	46g	29g	8g	4g	0g

INGREDIENTS

2 apples

4 tbsp oats

4 tbsp Greek yogurt

handful of blueberries

METHOD

01/ Grate apples and mix with the oats and Greek yogurt. Layer in a pot with blueberries.

Notes:

If the recipe doesn't fill you up enough, try adding some chopped or flaked almonds.

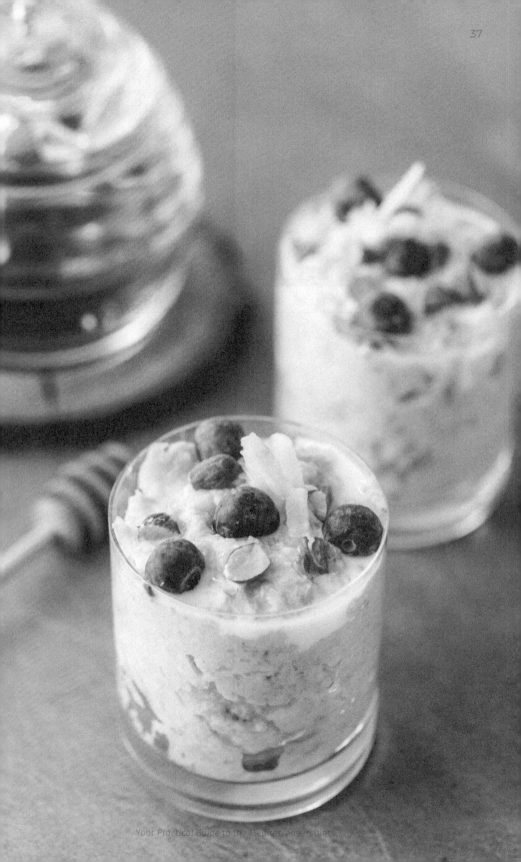

Blueberry Oats Bowl

SUITABLE
Vegetarian

PREP TIME
5 mins

COOK TIME
5 mins

SERVES
2

Nutrition (per serving)	Kcal	Fat	Sat Fat	Carb	Sugar	Fibre	Protein	Salt
	235	4g	1g	38g	14g	5g	13g	0.1g

INGREDIENTS

¾ cup / 60g porridge oats

⅔ up / 160g Greek yogurt

⅘ cup / 175g blueberries

1 tsp honey

METHOD

01/ Put the oats in a pan with 400ml of water. Heat and stir for about 2 minutes. Remove from the heat and add a third of the yogurt.

02/ Tip the blueberries into a pan with the honey and 1 tbsp of water. Gently poach until the blueberries are tender.

03/ Spoon the porridge into bowls and add the remaining yogurt and blueberries.

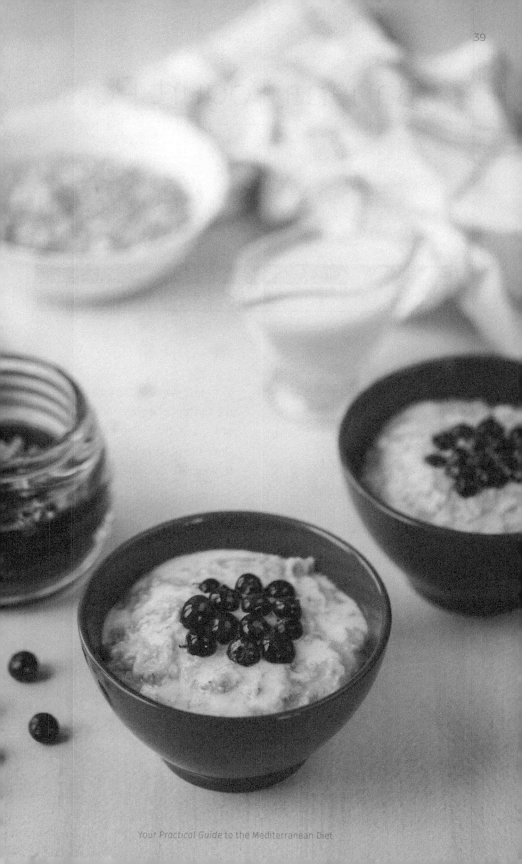

Banana Yogurt Pots

	SUITABLE	PREP TIME	COOK TIME	SERVES
	Vegetarian	5 mins	No Cook	2

Nutrition (per serving)	Kcal	Fat	Sat Fat	Carb	Sugar	Fibre	Protein	Salt
	236	7g	2g	32g	19g	4g	14g	0.1g

INGREDIENTS

1 cup / 225g Greek yogurt

2 bananas, sliced into chunks

2 tbsp / 15g walnuts, toasted and chopped

METHOD

01/ Place some of the yogurt into the bottom of a glass. Add a layer of banana, then yogurt and repeat. Once the glass is full, scatter with the nuts.

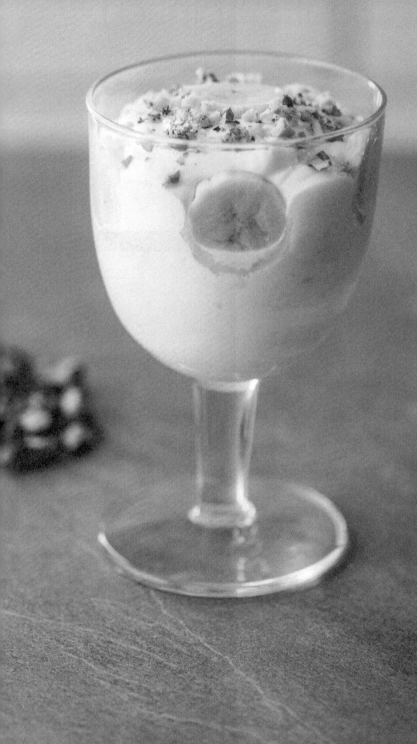

Basil & Spinach Scramble

SUITABLE
Vegetarian

PREP TIME
5 mins

COOK TIME
5 mins

SERVES
2

Nutrition (per serving)	Kcal	Fat	Sat Fat	Carb	Sugar	Fibre	Protein	Salt
	294	24g	5g	8g	4g	3g	16g	0.5g

INGREDIENTS

2 tbsp olive oil

⅔ cup / 100g cherry tomatoes

4 eggs

¼ cup / 60ml milk

handful basil, chopped

6 ⅔ cup / 200g baby spinach

black pepper

METHOD

01/ Heat 1 tbsp oil in a pan and add the tomatoes. While they are cooking, beat the eggs in a jug and add the milk, black pepper and basil.

02/ Remove the tomatoes from the pan and place on the plates. Add the oil, spinach and egg mixture to the pan, stirring occasionally until the eggs scramble. Once set, add to the plates and serve.

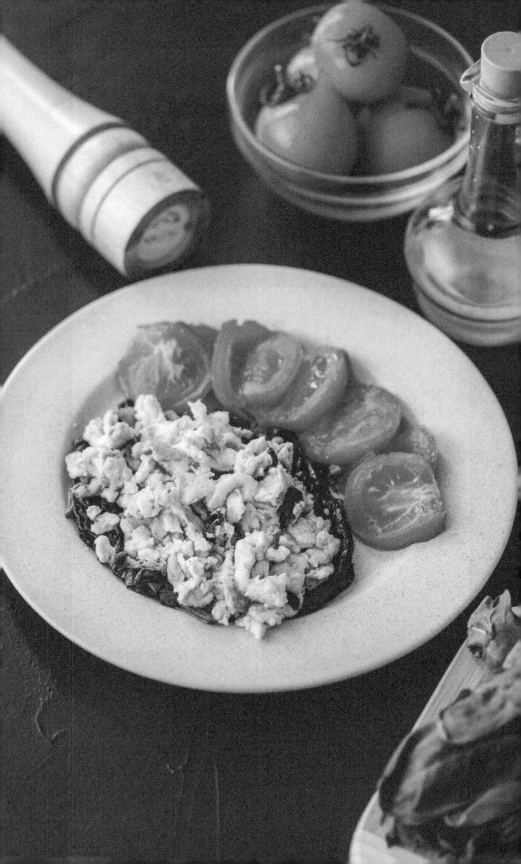

Fruity Bircher Muesli

SUITABLE
Vegetarian

PREP TIME
5 mins

COOK TIME
No Cook

SERVES
2

Nutrition (per serving)	Kcal	Fat	Sat Fat	Carb	Sugar	Fibre	Protein	Salt
	323	8g	2g	54g	24g	9g	12g	0.2g

INGREDIENTS

1 apple, coarsely grated

⅝ cup / 50g porridge oats

⅙ cup / 25g mixed seeds

½ tsp ground cinnamon

½ cup / 100g Greek yogurt

1 banana, sliced

1 tbsp / 10g raisins

METHOD

01/ Place the grated apple, oats, seeds and cinnamon into a bowl. Stir in the yogurt and 100ml of cold water, cover and leave in the fridge overnight.

02/ Spoon muesli into bowls and top with sliced bananas and raisins

Notes:

Try adding some chopped nuts such as almonds or walnuts.

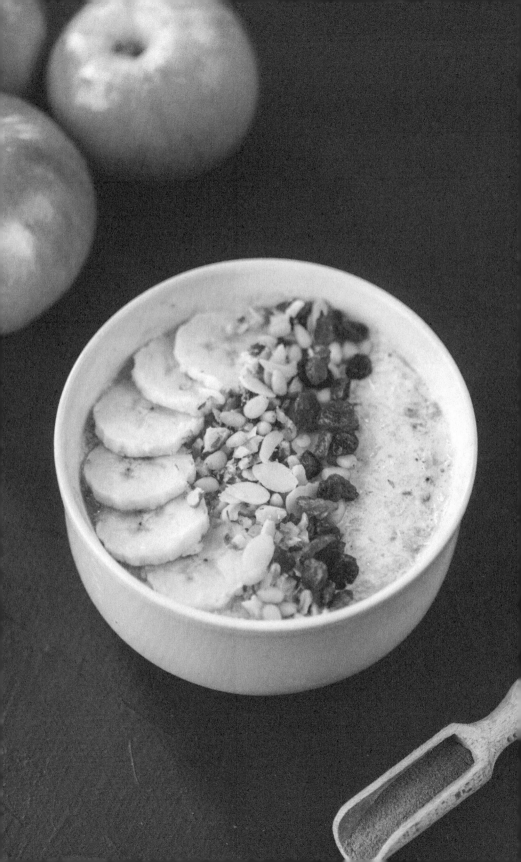

Strawberry & Almond Smoothie

SUITABLE
Vegetarian

PREP TIME
5 mins

COOK TIME
No Cook

SERVES
2

Nutrition (per serving)	Kcal	Fat	Sat Fat	Carb	Sugar	Fibre	Protein	Salt
	239	9g	1g	36g	19g	6g	8g	0.1g

INGREDIENTS

2 bananas

8 strawberries

⅕ cup / 50g Greek yogurt

⅕ up / 50ml milk

¼ cup / 30g ground almonds

METHOD

01/ Slice the banana into a blender and add strawberries, yogurt, milk and ground almonds. Blitz until completely smooth.

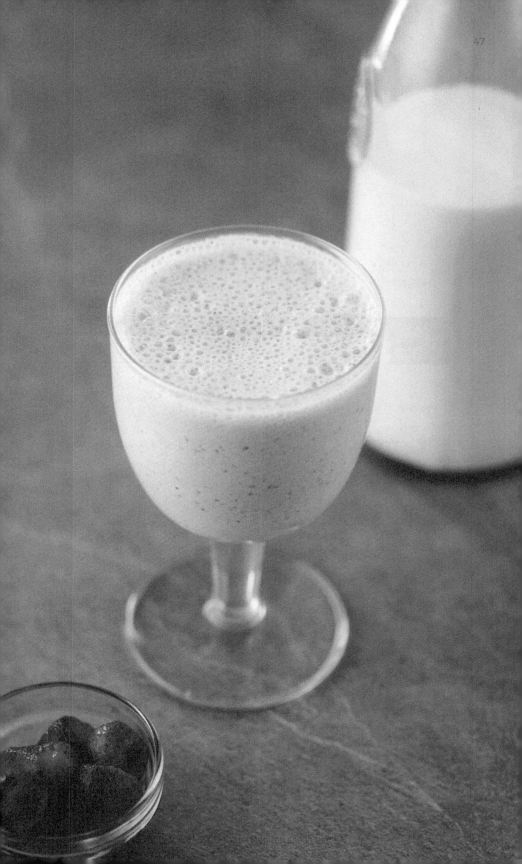

Veggie Stir Fry Omelette

SUITABLE
Vegetarian

PREP TIME
5 mins

COOK TIME
5 mins

SERVES
2

Nutrition (per serving)	Kcal	Fat	Sat Fat	Carb	Sugar	Fibre	Protein	Salt
	194	13g	3g	6g	3g	2g	12g	0.6g

INGREDIENTS

4 eggs

2 tsp olive oil

5-6 oz / 160g vegetable stir fry mix

1 tsp reduced-salt soy sauce

METHOD

01/ Beat the eggs and season. Heat the olive oil in a pan, add the stir fry vegetable mix and cook until tender, then add soy sauce.

02/ Pour in the eggs and cook until they are lightly set, then serve.

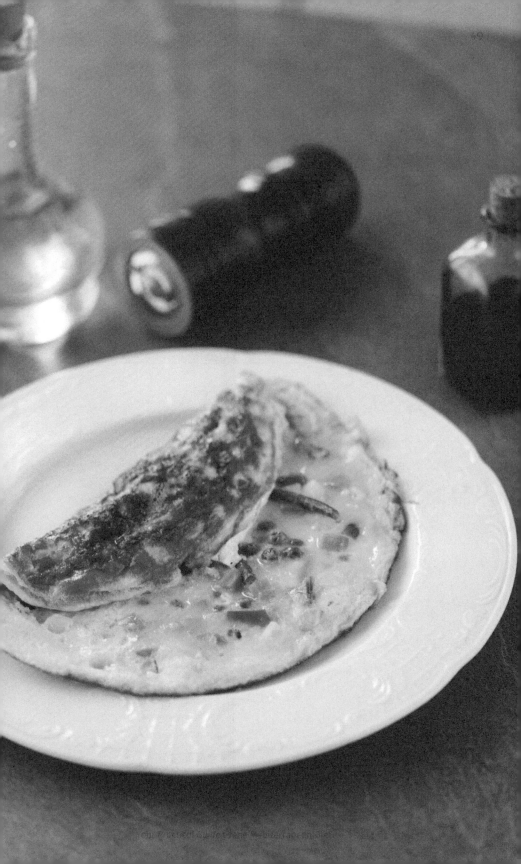

Tomato & Watermelon Salad

———

SUITABLE
Vegetarian

PREP TIME
5 mins

COOK TIME
No Cook

SERVES
2

Nutrition (per serving)	Kcal	Fat	Sat Fat	Carb	Sugar	Fibre	Protein	Salt
	177	13g	5g	13g	10g	1g	5g	0.7g

INGREDIENTS

1 tbsp olive oil

1 tbsp red wine vinegar

¼ tsp chilli flakes

1 tbsp chopped mint

⅘ cup / 120g tomatoes, chopped

1 ½ cups / 250g watermelon, cut into chunks

⅔ cup / 100g feta cheese, crumbled

METHOD

01/ For the dressing, Mix the oil, vinegar, chilli flakes and mint and then season.

02/ Put the tomatoes and watermelon into a bowl. Pour over the dressing, add the feta, then serve.

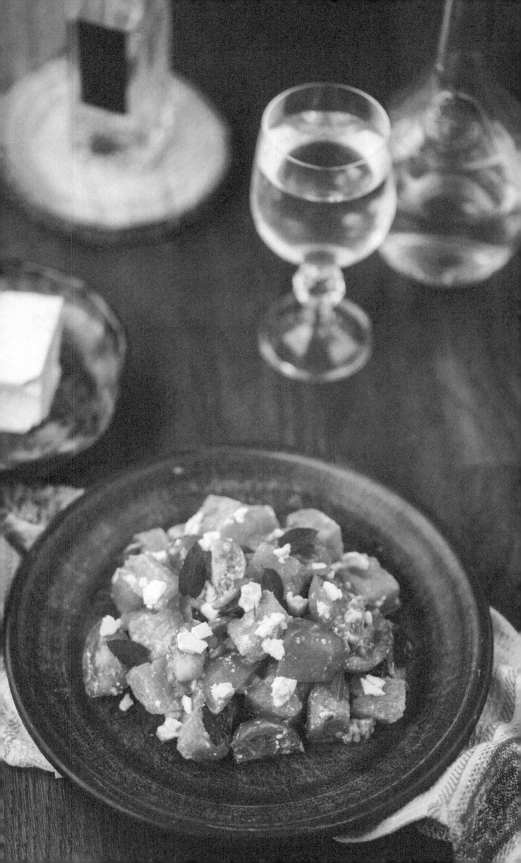

Kiwi Yogurt with Chia Seeds

SUITABLE
Vegan

PREP TIME
10 mins

COOK TIME
No Cook

SERVES
2

Nutrition (per serving)	Kcal	Fat	Sat Fat	Carb	Sugar	Fibre	Protein	Salt
	360	12g	6g	57g	28g	10g	9g	0.01g

INGREDIENTS

2 kiwis, peeled and sliced

1 banana, sliced

½ up / 100g blueberries

1 tbsp chia seeds

3 tbsp granola

2 figs, chopped

3 dried apple rings, chopped

½ cup / 200g soya yogurt

1 tsp honey

METHOD

01/ Mix the yogurt and honey together and divide between two bowls. Place the banana, blueberries, kiwis and chia seeds on top of the yogurt. Sprinkle over the figs, dried apple rings and granola. Serve immediately.

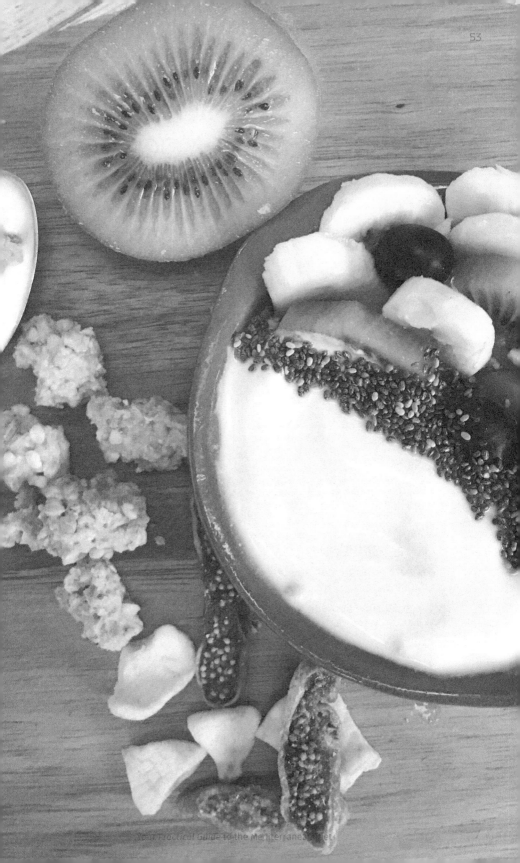

French Toast Muffins & Blueberry Yogurt

SUITABLE

Vegetarian

PREP TIME

10 mins

COOK TIME

5 mins

SERVES

2

Nutrition (per serving)	Kcal	Fat	Sat Fat	Carb	Sugar	Fibre	Protein	Salt
	300	14g	3g	30g	24g	2g	14g	0.2g

INGREDIENTS

1 tsbp olive oil

2 muffins

2 eggs

⅖ cup / 100ml milk

2 tsp honey

⅖ cup / 100g Greek yogurt

1 tbsp hazelnuts, toasted and chopped

¾ cup / 150g blueberries

METHOD

01 / Whisk the milk and egg together and split open the muffins. Soak each half in the egg mix.

02 / Heat the oil in a frying pan. Toast the eggy muffin halves until crisp on the outside and soft in the center..

03 / Mix the berries, yogurt and honey.

04 / Place muffins on plates. Top with blueberry yogurt, scatter with hazelnuts and serve.

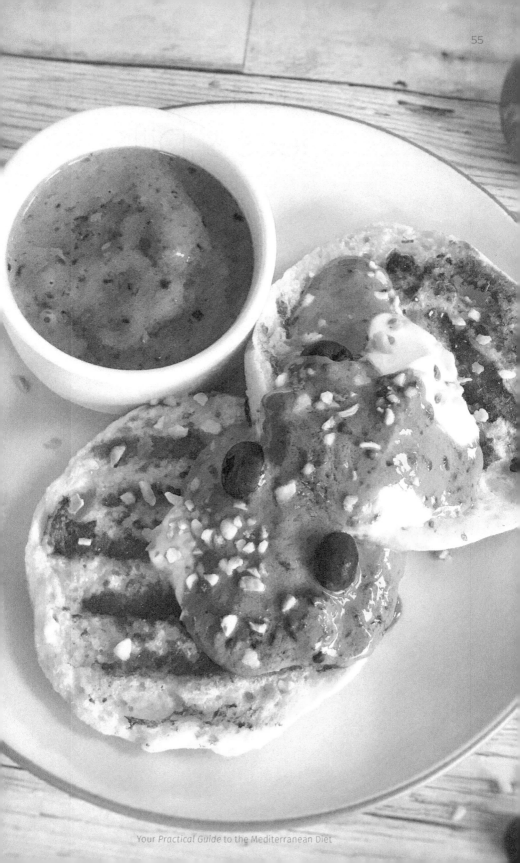

Avocado Toast with Seeds & Dill

SUITABLE

Vegan

PREP TIME

5 mins

COOK TIME

No Cook

SERVES

2

Nutrition (per serving)	Kcal	Fat	Sat Fat	Carb	Sugar	Fibre	Protein	Salt
	344	18g	3g	37g	5g	7g	14g	0.6g

INGREDIENTS

2 slices of wholemeal bread

1 avocado

2 spring onions, sliced

1 tbsp pumpkin or sesame seeds

handful of plum tomatoes, sliced

2 sprigs of dill, roughly chopped

METHOD

01/ Lightly toast the bread. Meanwhile, halve the avocado, remove the stone and scoop out the flesh. Mash the avocado and mix in half of the dill.

02/ Spread the avocado on the toast, layer on the tomatoes and sprinkle over the seeds, spring onions and remaining dill, then serve.

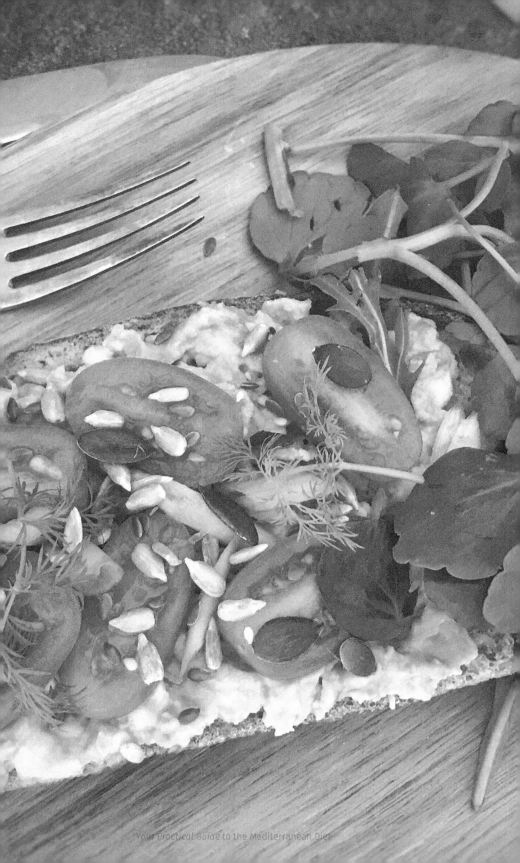

Smoked Mackerel & Lemon Rice

SUITABLE
Quick

PREP TIME
5 mins

COOK TIME
5 mins

SERVES
2

Nutrition (per serving)	Kcal	Fat	Sat Fat	Carb	Sugar	Fibre	Protein	Salt
	456	18g	5g	54g	3g	6g	20g	0.2g

INGREDIENTS

1 tsp olive oil

1 hard-boiled egg, chopped

1 ½ cups / 250g ready cooked basmati rice pouch

½ onion, finely chopped

1 lemon, zest only

1 tsp mild curry powder

2 smoked mackerel fillets, flaked

1 tsp dried oregano

pea shoots, to serve

METHOD

01/ Heat the oil in a saucepan. Add the onion and stir for 3-4 minutes, until soft. Add the curry spice and stir for a further minute. Add the basmati rice to the saucepan and stir well until heated thoroughly.

02/ Add the lemon and the mackerel and stir until heated through.

03/ Divide the rice and mackerel mixture between 2 bowls and scatter over the egg. Serve with pea shoots

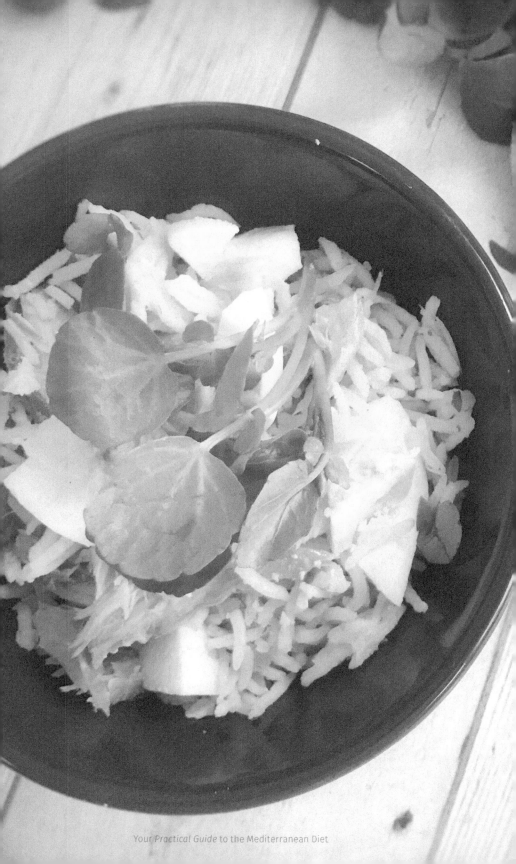

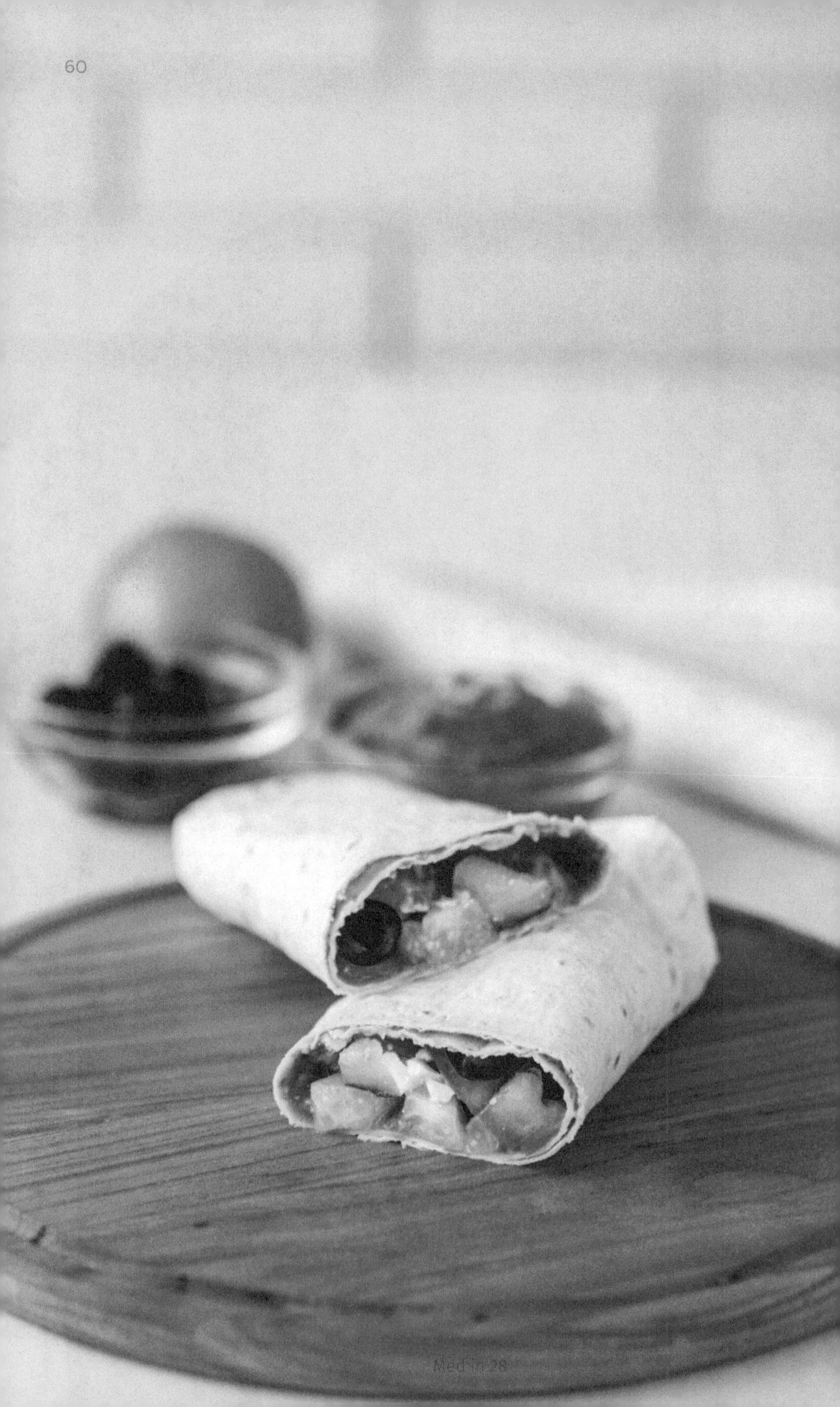

Lunch

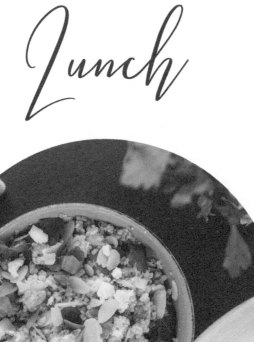

Mixed Bean Salad

SUITABLE
Vegetarian

PREP TIME
10 mins

COOK TIME
No Cook

SERVES
2

Nutrition (per serving)	Kcal	Fat	Sat Fat	Carb	Sugar	Fibre	Protein	Salt
	240	12g	5g	22g	4g	9g	11g	1.5g

INGREDIENTS

1 cup / 145g jar artichoke heart in oil

½ tbsp sundried tomato paste

½ tsp red wine vinegar

1 x 7oz can / 200g can cannellini beans, drained and rinsed

1 cup / 150g cherry tomatoes, quartered

handful Kalamata black olives

2 spring onions, thinly sliced on the diagonal

⅔ cup / 100g feta cheese, crumbled

METHOD

01 / Drain the jar of artichokes, reserving 1-2 tbsp of oil. Add the oil, sun-dried tomato paste and vinegar and stir until smooth. Season to taste.

02 / Chop the artichokes and tip into a bowl. Add the cannellini beans, tomatoes, olives, spring onions and half of the feta cheese. Stir in the artichoke oil mixture and tip into a serving bowl. Crumble over the remaining feta cheese, then serve.

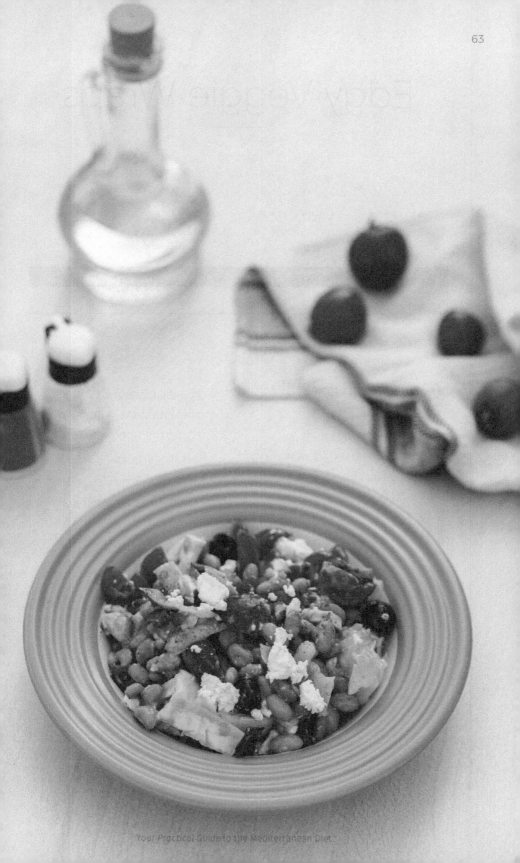

Edgy Veggie Wraps

SUITABLE
Vegetarian

PREP TIME
10 mins

COOK TIME
No Cook

SERVES
2

Nutrition (per serving)	Kcal	Fat	Sat Fat	Carb	Sugar	Fibre	Protein	Salt
	310	11g	5g	39g	6g	8g	11g	1.6g

INGREDIENTS

⅔ cup / 100g cherry tomato

1 cucumber

6 kalamata olives

2 large wholemeal tortilla wraps

⅓ up / 50g feta cheese

2 tbsp hummus

METHOD

01 / Chop the tomatoes, cut the cucumber into sticks, split the olives and remove the stones.

02 / Heat the tortillas.

03 / Spread the hummus over the wrap. Put the vegetable mix in the middle and roll up.

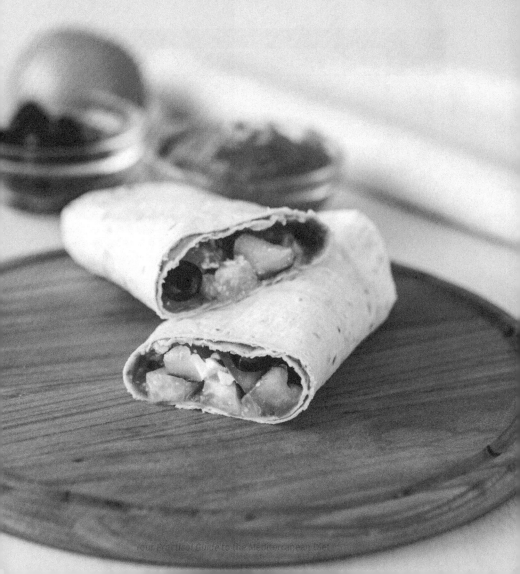

Speedy Couscous Salad

SUITABLE
Vegetarian

PREP TIME
10 mins

COOK TIME
No Cook

SERVES
2

Nutrition (per serving)	Kcal	Fat	Sat Fat	Carb	Sugar	Fibre	Protein	Salt
	395	16g	6g	51g	8g	5g	14g	1.8g

INGREDIENTS

½ cup / 100g couscous

1 cup / 200ml vegetable stock

2 spring onions

1 red pepper

½ cucumber

⅓ cup / 50g feta cheese, cubed

2 tbsp pesto

2 tbsp toasted almonds

METHOD

01/ Pour couscous into a bowl and pour in the stock. Cover the bowl, then leave for 10 minutes, until the stock is absorbed.

02/ In the meantime, slice the onions and pepper and dice the cucumber. Add these to the couscous and fork in the pesto. Crumble the feta, then sprinkle over the toasted almonds to serve.

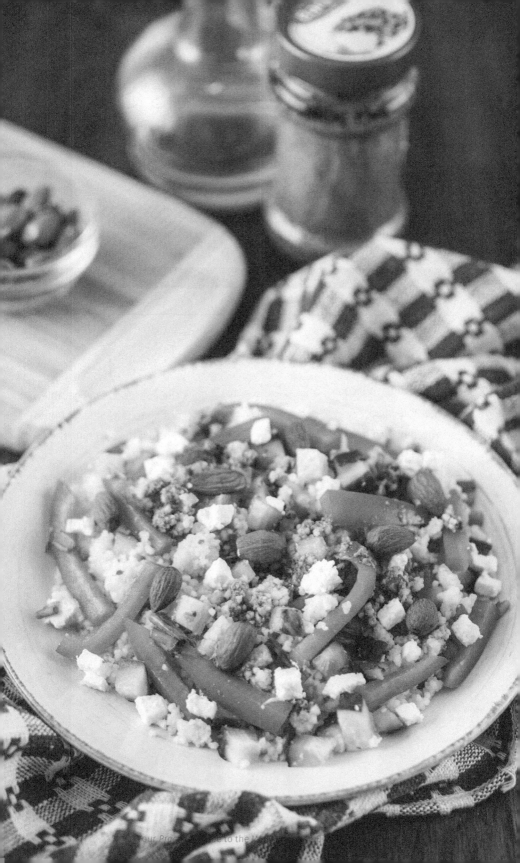

Tangy Couscous Salad

SUITABLE
Vegetarian

PREP TIME
5 mins

COOK TIME
10 mins

SERVES
2

Nutrition (per serving)	Kcal	Fat	Sat Fat	Carb	Sugar	Fibre	Protein	Salt
	353	14g	6g	48g	6g	5g	12g	1.6g

INGREDIENTS

1 cup / 200g couscous

vegetable stock

2 zucchini / courgettes

1 tbsp olive oil

⅓ cup / 50g feta cheese, crumbled

¾ cup / 20g parsley, chopped

juice 1 lemon

METHOD

01/ Cook the couscous in vegetable stock according to pack instructions. Trim the ends off the zucchini, then cut into slices.

02/ Heat the oil in a pan. Add the zucchini and season. Cook for 2 minutes, then turn over and cook until soft. Tip into a large bowl along with the cooked couscous. Add remaining ingredients, mix through and serve.

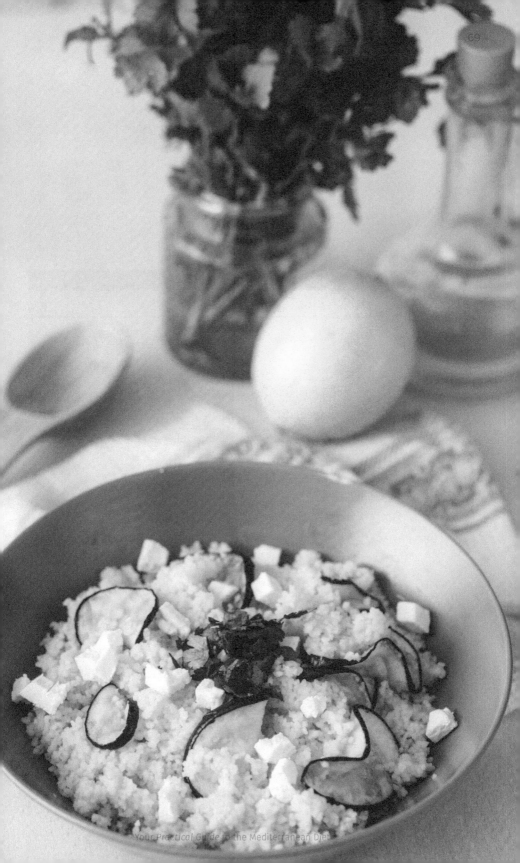

Greek Salad

SUITABLE
Vegetarian

PREP TIME
5 mins

COOK TIME
No Cook

SERVES
2

Nutrition (per serving)	Kcal	Fat	Sat Fat	Carb	Sugar	Fibre	Protein	Salt
	273	24g	6g	14g	6g	4g	6g	1.5g

INGREDIENTS

⅘ cup / 120g tomatoes, quartered

1 cucumber, peeled, deseeded, then roughly chopped

½ red onion, thinly sliced

16 Kalamata olives

1 tsp dried oregano

⅓ cup / 50g feta cheese, crumbled

2 tbsp olive oil

METHOD

01/ Place all of the ingredients in a large bowl and lightly season. Serve with wholemeal bread.

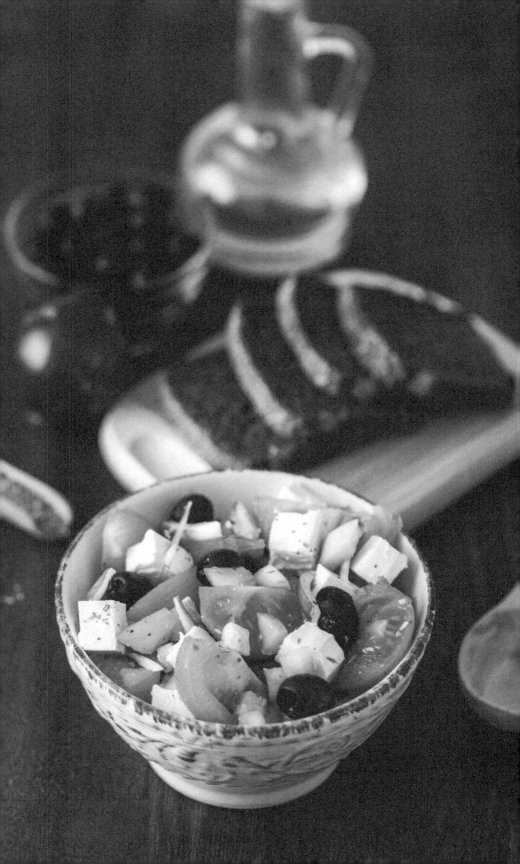

Cannellini Bean Salad

SUITABLE

Vegan

PREP TIME

5 mins

COOK TIME

No Cook

SERVES

2

Nutrition (per serving)	Kcal	Fat	Sat Fat	Carb	Sugar	Fibre	Protein	Salt
	302	0g	0g	54g	5g	25g	20g	1.2g

INGREDIENTS

1 x 21 oz / 600g can cannellini beans

½ cup / 70g cherry tomatoes, halved

½ red onion, thinly sliced

½ tbsp red wine vinegar

small bunch basil, torn

METHOD

01/ Rinse and drain the beans and mix with the tomatoes, onion and vinegar. Season, then add basil just before serving.

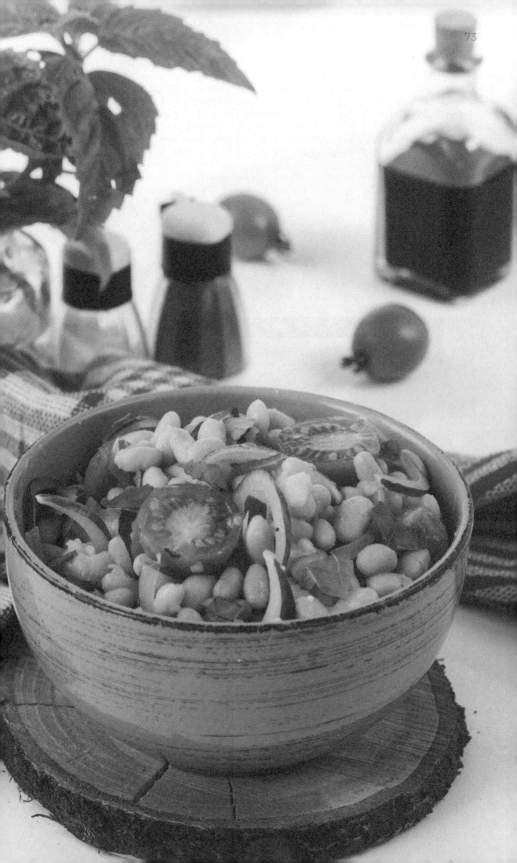

Carrot, Orange & Avocado Salad

SUITABLE
Vegan

PREP TIME
10 mins

COOK TIME
No Cook

SERVES
2

Nutrition (per serving)	Kcal	Fat	Sat Fat	Carb	Sugar	Fibre	Protein	Salt
	338	27g	5g	26g	13g	11g	4g	0.1g

INGREDIENTS

1 orange, plus zest and juice of 1

2 carrots, halved lengthways and sliced with a peeler

⅓ cup / 35g rocket /arugula

1 avocado, stoned, peeled and sliced

1 tbsp olive oil

METHOD

01/ Cut the segments from 1 of the oranges and put in a bowl with the carrots, arugula and avocado. Whisk together the orange juice, zest and oil. Toss through the salad, and season.

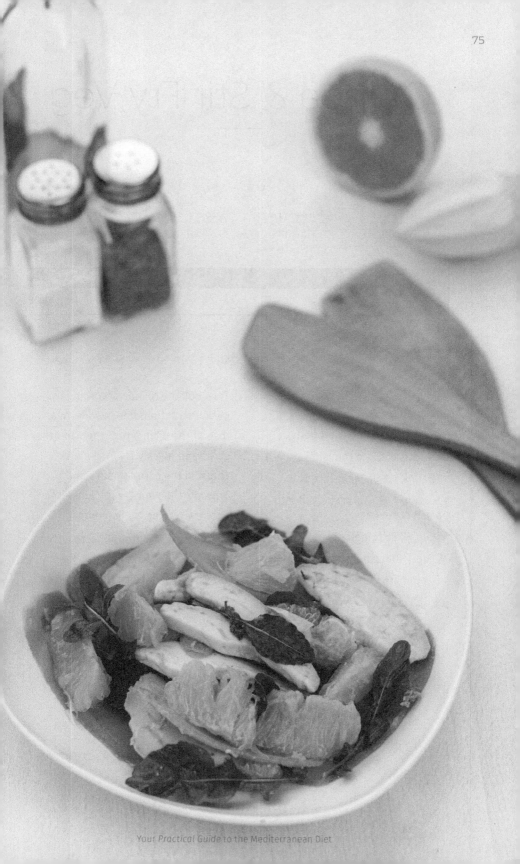

Quinoa & Stir Fry Veg

SUITABLE

Vegan

PREP TIME

15 mins

COOK TIME

15 mins

SERVES

2

Nutrition (per serving)	Kcal	Fat	Sat Fat	Carb	Sugar	Fibre	Protein	Salt
	473	25g	3g	56g	9g	9g	11g	0.3g

INGREDIENTS

½ cup/ 100g quinoa

3 tbsp olive oil

1 garlic clove, finely chopped

2 carrots, cut into thin sticks

1 ½ cups / 150g leek, sliced

1 ½ cups / 150g broccoli, cut into
  small florets

¼ cup / 50g tomatoes

⅖ cup / 100ml vegetable stock

1 tsp tomato purée

juice ½ lemon

METHOD

01 / Cook the quinoa according to pack instructions. Meanwhile, heat 3 tbsp of the oil in a pan, then add the garlic and quickly fry for 1 minute. Throw in the carrots, leeks and broccoli, then stir-fry for 2 minutes until everything is glistening.

02 / Add the tomatoes, mix together the stock and tomato purée, then add to the pan. Cover and cook for 3 minutes. Drain the quinoa and toss in the remaining oil and lemon juice. Divide between warm plates and spoon the vegetables on top.

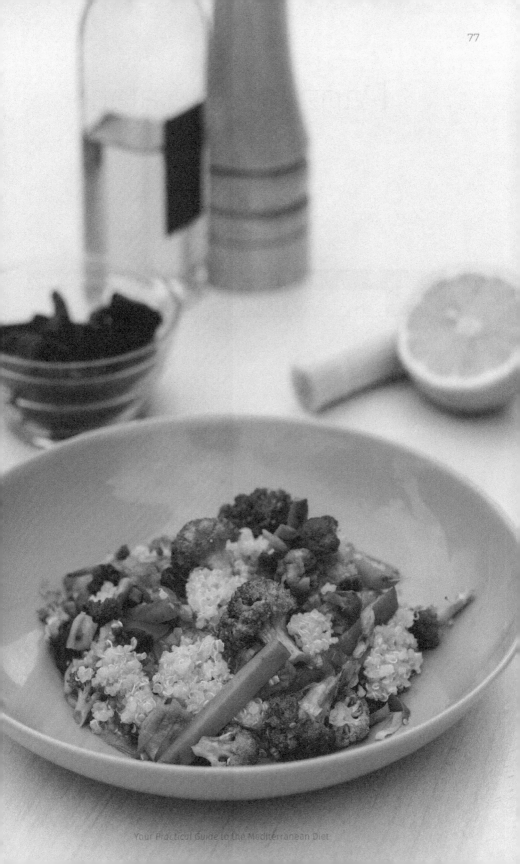

Panzanella Salad

SUITABLE
Vegan

PREP TIME
20 mins

COOK TIME
No Cook

SERVES
2

Nutrition (per serving)	Kcal	Fat	Sat Fat	Carb	Sugar	Fibre	Protein	Salt
	452	35g	6g	37g	7g	11g	6g	1.1g

INGREDIENTS

2 ⅔ cups / 400g tomatoes

1 garlic clove, crushed

1 tbsp capers, drained and rinsed

1 ripe avocado, stoned, peeled and chopped

1 small red onion, very thinly sliced

2 slices of brown bread

2 tbsp olive oil

1 tbsp red wine vinegar

small handful basil leaves

METHOD

01/ Chop the tomatoes and put them in a bowl. Season well and add the garlic, capers, avocado and onion. Mix well and set aside for 10 minutes.

02/ Meanwhile, tear the bread into chunks and place in a bowl. Drizzle over half of the olive oil and half of the vinegar. When ready to serve, scatter tomatoes and basil leaves and drizzle with remaining oil and vinegar. Stir before serving.

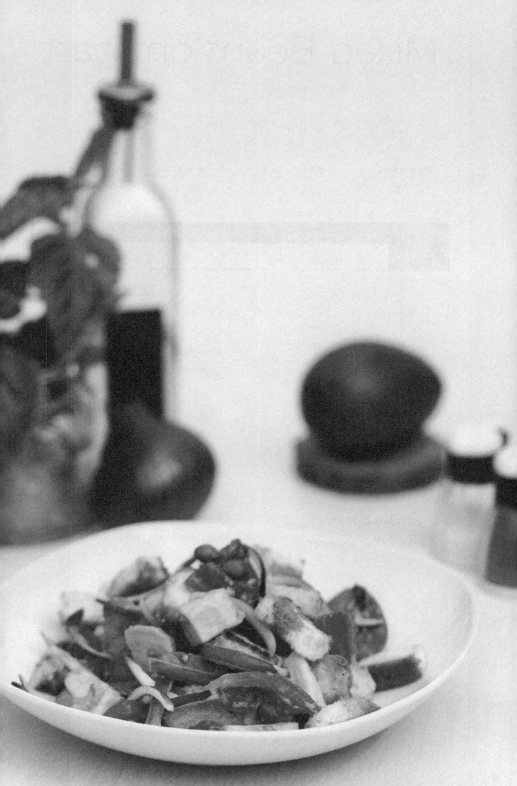

Mixed Beans on Toast

SUITABLE
Vegan

PREP TIME
5 mins

COOK TIME
5 mins

SERVES
2

Nutrition (per serving)	Kcal	Fat	Sat Fat	Carb	Sugar	Fibre	Protein	Salt
	261	2g	0g	49g	8g	15g	13g	1.3g

INGREDIENTS

1 onion, halved and sliced

½ red bell pepper, sliced

1 tsp olive oil

1 tsp smoked sweet paprika

½ tin of tomatoes

½ tin of chickpeas

½ tin of cannellini beans

handful of spinach

2 slices of brown bread

coriander / cilantro, to serve

METHOD

01/ In a saucepan, heat the oil. Add the onion and pepper and stir for 3-4 minutes, until soft. Add the tomatoes, salt and paprika and stir well.

02/ While simmering, add the spinach, chickpeas and beans and heat until piping hot and the spinach wilted.

03/ Toast the bread and serve the beans between two plates and top with cilantro.

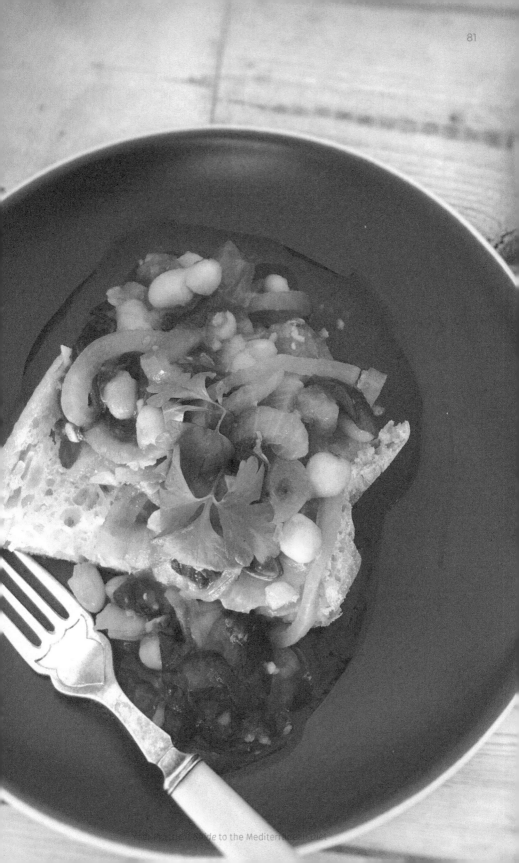

Prawn & Ratatouille Omelette

SUITABLE
Quick

PREP TIME
5 mins

COOK TIME
5 mins

SERVES
2

Nutrition (per serving)	Kcal	Fat	Sat Fat	Carb	Sugar	Fibre	Protein	Salt
	461	23g	6g	39g	8g	6g	23g	0.7g

INGREDIENTS

2 tsp olive oil

½ onion, chopped finely

1 green bell pepper, sliced

1 garlic clove, crushed

½ tin of tomatoes

Handful of cooked prawns

6 eggs, beaten

salt and pepper

mixed salad to serve

METHOD

01/ In a saucepan, heat 1 tsp of the oil. Add the onion and garlic and stir for 3-4 minutes, until soft. Add the pepper and tomatoes and cook until simmering. Stir through the prawns.

02/ Heat the remaining oil in a saucepan. When really hot, add half of the egg mix. Swirl around the pan until the bottom of the omelette begins to set. Cook until lightly set and tip half of the prawn mix on to one half of the omelette. Fold over and place on a heated plate and keep warm. Repeat with the remaining ingredients.

03/ Plate the omelettes and add the mixed salad. Serve immediately.

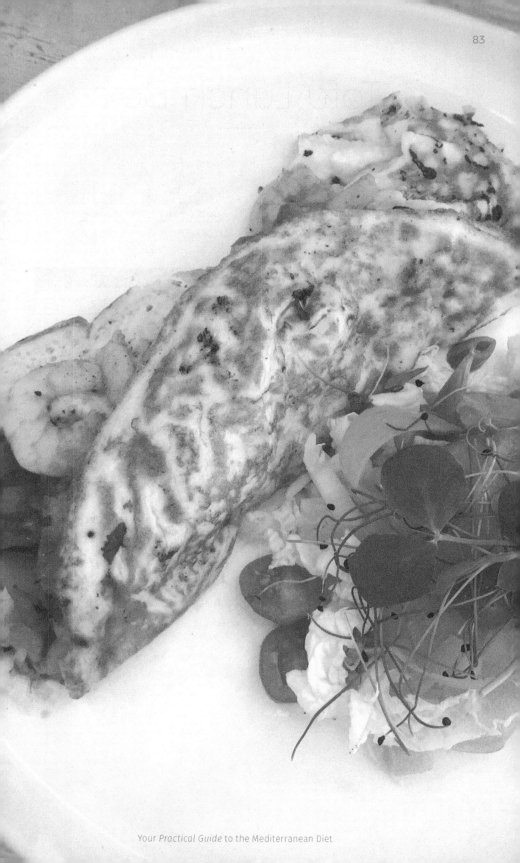

Tofu Lunch Box

SUITABLE
Vegan

PREP TIME
5 mins

COOK TIME
10 mins

SERVES
2

Nutrition (per serving)	Kcal	Fat	Sat Fat	Carb	Sugar	Fibre	Protein	Salt
	445	10g	1g	53g	11g	10g	19g	0.7g

INGREDIENTS

3 tbsp honey

3 tbsp lemon juice

1 tsp garlic powder

1 tsp olive oil

⅘ cup / 200g tofu, firm, drained and pressed

1 medium carrot, shredded with a ribbon peeler

1 pepper, sliced

handful of rocket /arugula

1 tbsp sesame seeds

1 ½ cups / 250g ready cooked quinoa

METHOD

01/ Cut the tofu into cubes and mix with honey, garlic powder and lemon juice. Leave to one side for 1 hour, or leave in the fridge for up to 24 hours.

02/ Heat the oil in a saucepan and add the cubes of tofu. Cook over a high heat to produce crusty, golden sides. Leave to cool.

03/ Mix the rest of the ingredients together and stir through the cooled tofu. Drizzle with dressing just before serving.

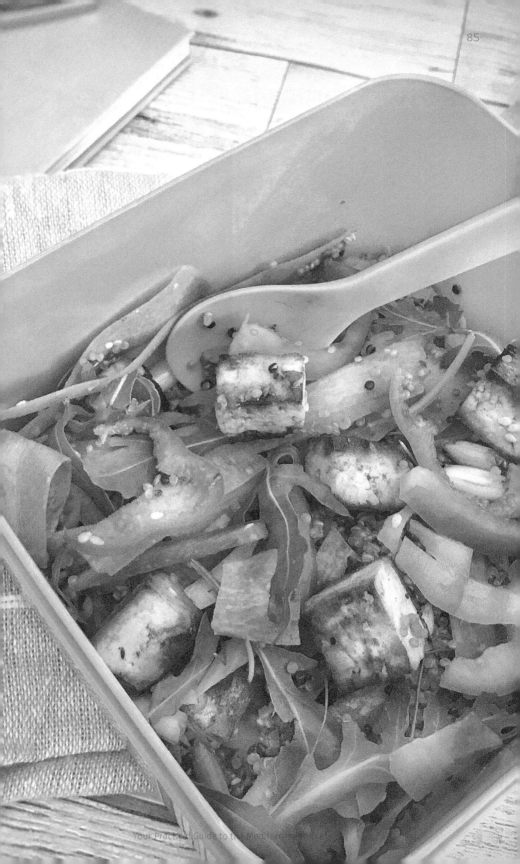

Moroccan Chickpea Soup

SUITABLE

Vegan

PREP TIME

5 mins

COOK TIME

20 mins

SERVES

2

Nutrition (per serving)	Kcal	Fat	Sat Fat	Carb	Sugar	Fibre	Protein	Salt
	408	11g	2g	63g	3g	10g	15g	2.0g

INGREDIENTS

1 tbsp olive oil

½ medium onion, chopped

1 celery sticks, chopped

1 tsp ground cumin

1 ⅕ cups / 300ml hot vegetable stock

7 oz / 200g can chopped tomatoes

7 oz / 200g can chickpeas, rinsed and drained

½ cup / 50g frozen broad beans

zest and juice ½ lemon

coriander / cilantro & bread to serve

METHOD

01/ Heat the oil in a saucepan, then fry the onion and celery for 10 minutes until softened. Add the cumin and fry for another minute.

02/ Turn up the heat, then add the stock, tomatoes, chickpeas and black pepper. Simmer for 8 minutes. Add broad beans and lemon juice and cook for a further 2 minutes. Top with lemon zest and cilantro.

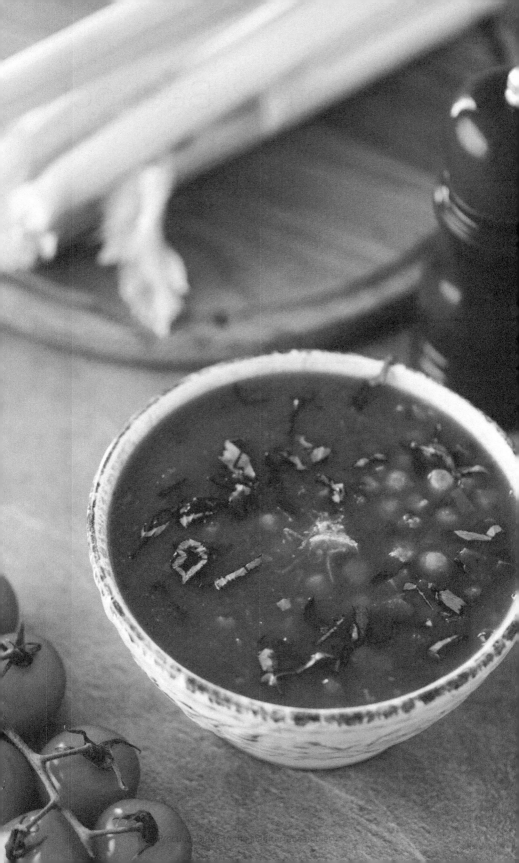

Mackerel & Beetroot Wrap

SUITABLE
Quick

PREP TIME
5 mins

COOK TIME
5 mins

SERVES
2

Nutrition (per serving)	Kcal	Fat	Sat Fat	Carb	Sugar	Fibre	Protein	Salt
	461	23g	6g	39g	8g	5g	23g	0.7g

INGREDIENTS

- 2 wholemeal wraps
- 1 smoked mackerel fillet, flaked
- 1 small beetroot, raw, peeled and grated
- 1-2 tsp of walnuts
- 2 tbsp black beans
- 1-2 tsp mixed seeds
- 2 tbsp Greek yogurt
- 2 handfuls of rocket / arugula

METHOD

01/ On two plates, lay the tortilla wraps. Divide the arugula over the middle of each. Scatter the beetroot over the arugula. Divide the mackerel flakes over the beetroot. Add the beans on both piles.

02/ Place a spoonful of the yoghurt on top and sprinkle over the seeds and nuts.

03/ Roll up, cut up, or eat as you wish!

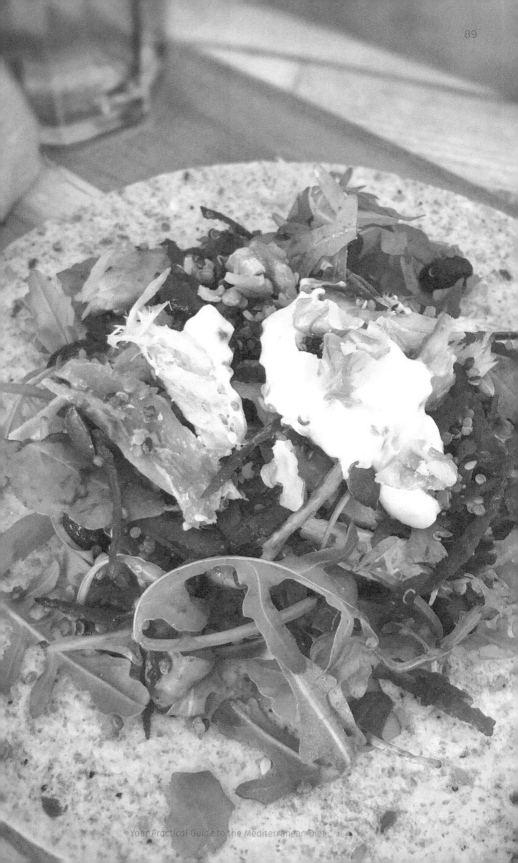

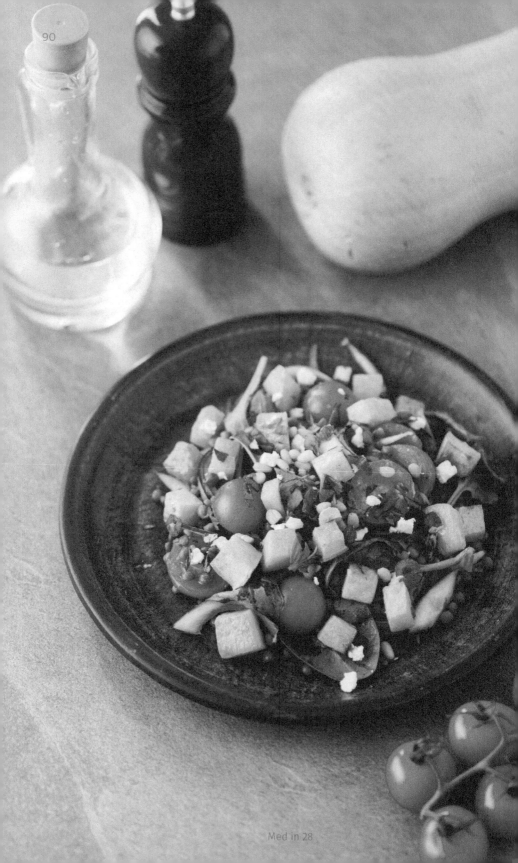

Dinner

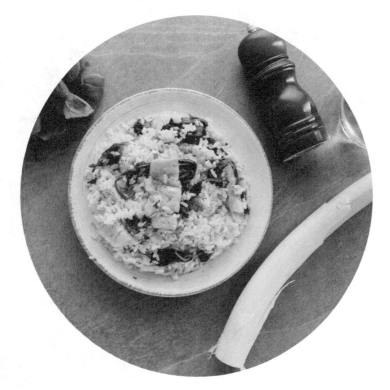

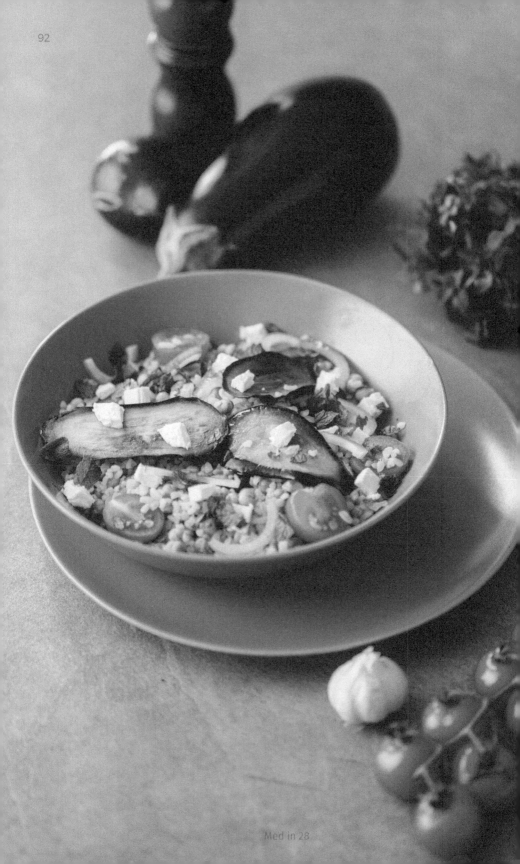

Vegetarian

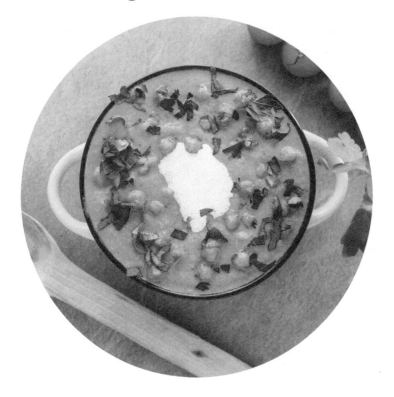

Spinach Spaghetti

SUITABLE

Quick

PREP TIME

5 mins

COOK TIME

15 mins

SERVES

2

Nutrition (per serving)	Kcal	Fat	Sat Fat	Carb	Sugar	Fibre	Protein	Salt
	425	25g	5g	42g	3g	10g	15g	0.6g

INGREDIENTS

1 ¼ cups / 250g pack wholewheat spaghetti

8 cups / 250g spinach

1-2 tbsp olive oil, plus extra to serve

2 garlic cloves, finely sliced

1 tbsp red wine vinegar

handful almonds

⅙ cup / 25g feta

chilli flakes, to serve

METHOD

01/ Cook the spaghetti according to pack instructions. Meanwhile, boil the kettle & place the spinach into a colander and pour over boiling water until it's wilted. Cool under cold water and squeeze into a ball until the water has been removed.

02/ Gently heat oil and garlic in a pan until it just starts to brown, then add vinegar. Simmer for 1 minute, then turn off the heat. Drain the spaghetti once cooked. Toss in the oil, spinach, almonds and feta. Add chilli flakes and drizzle with olive oil to serve.

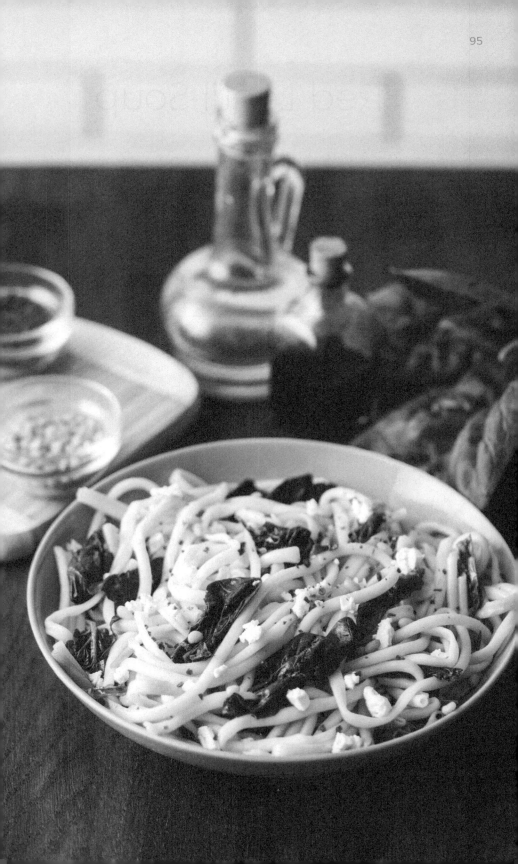

Red Lentil Soup

SUITABLE
/

PREP TIME
10 mins

COOK TIME
25 mins

SERVES
4

Nutrition (per serving)	Kcal	Fat	Sat Fat	Carb	Sugar	Fibre	Protein	Salt
	315	8g	4g	41g	11g	15g	24g	2.3g

INGREDIENTS

2 tsp cumin seed

large pinch chilli flakes

1 tbsp olive oil

1 red onion, chopped

¾ 140g red split lentils

3 ½ cups / 850ml vegetable stock

14 oz / 400g can tomatoes, chopped

7 oz / 200g can chickpeas, rinsed
  and drained

small bunch of coriander / cilantro

4 tbsp Greek yogurt

METHOD

01/ Heat a saucepan and fry the cumin seeds & chilli flakes for 1 minute. Add the oil and onion and cook for 5 minutes. Stir in the lentils, stock and tomatoes, then bring to the boil. Simmer for 15 minutes until the lentils have softened.

02/ Whizz the soup with a hand blender until it is a rough purée, pour back into the pan and add the chickpeas. Heat gently, season well and add cilantro and Greek yogurt to finish.

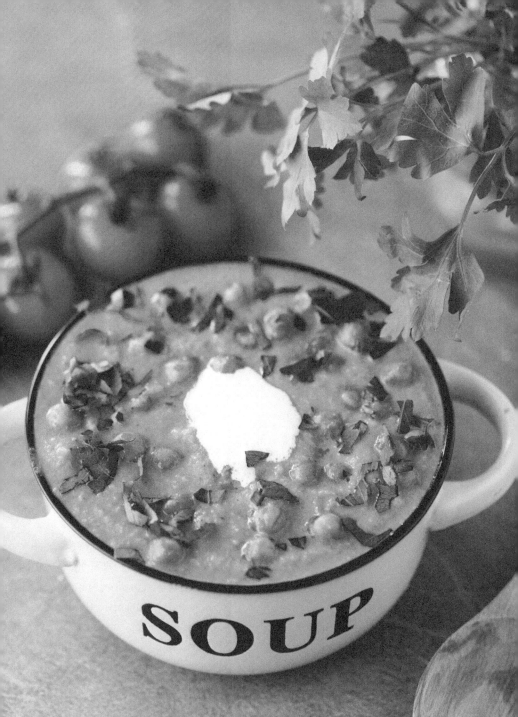

Grilled Eggplant & Tabbouleh

SUITABLE

Quick

PREP TIME

10 mins

COOK TIME

20 mins

SERVES

2

Nutrition (per serving)	Kcal	Fat	Sat Fat	Carb	Sugar	Fibre	Protein	Salt
	424	21g	6g	50g	11g	17g	13g	1.5g

INGREDIENTS

⅓ cup / 70g bulgur wheat

1 garlic clove, crushed

2 tbsp olive oil

1 eggplant / aubergine, thinly sliced

7 oz / 200g can chickpeas, drained

½ cup / 70g cherry tomatoes, halved

½ red onion, chopped

⅓ cup / 50g feta cheese, crumbled

bunch of mint, leaves chopped

juice of 1 lemon

METHOD

01 / Cook the bulgur wheat according to pack instructions, then drain well. In a bowl, mix the garlic and olive oil and drizzle some of the olive oil over both sides of the eggplant strips. Sear the strips in a frying pan for 3 minutes each side until charred.

02 / Tip the bulgur wheat into a bowl with the chickpeas, tomatoes, onion, feta & mint, then pour over the remaining oil and lemon juice. Mix & season well, then serve with eggplant.

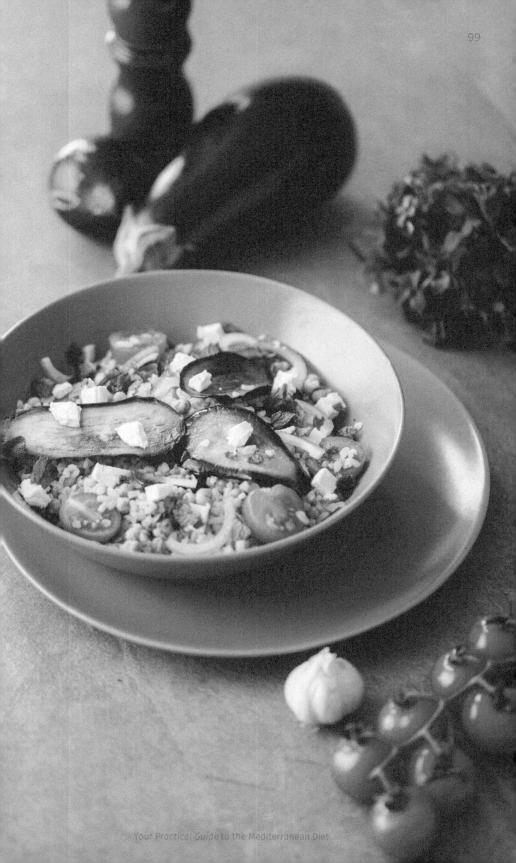

Greek Salad Omelette

SUITABLE
Quick

PREP TIME
5 mins

COOK TIME
20 mins

SERVES
2

Nutrition (per serving)	Kcal	Fat	Sat Fat	Carb	Sugar	Fibre	Protein	Salt
	369	21g	8g	10g	3g	1g	15g	2.3g

INGREDIENTS

4 eggs

handful of parsley leaves, chopped

1 tbsp olive oil

½ large red onion

⅔ cup / 100g cherry tomato,

handful black olives

⅓ cup / 50g feta cheese, crumbled

METHOD

01/ Heat the grill to high. Whisk the eggs in a bowl with the chopped parsley, pepper and salt. Heat the oil in a frying pan, then fry the onion over a high heat for about 4 minutes until they start to brown. Add the tomatoes and olives and cook for about 2 minutes.

02/ Turn the heat to medium & add the eggs, cooking them for about 2 minutes, stirring until they begin to set. Add feta, then place the pan under the grill for 5-6 minutes until the omelette is golden. Cut into wedges and serve.

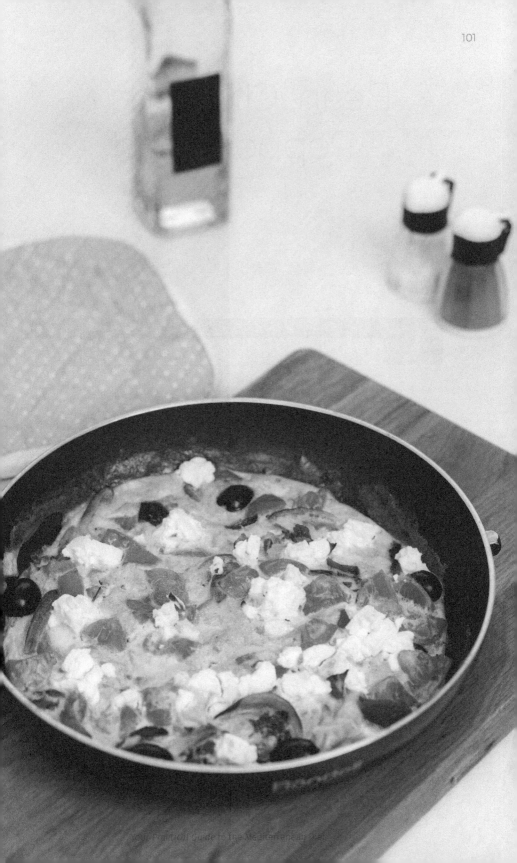

Bean, Chickpea & Pepper Salad

SUITABLE
Quick

PREP TIME
5 mins

COOK TIME
10 mins

SERVES
2

Nutrition (per serving)	Kcal	Fat	Sat Fat	Carb	Sugar	Fibre	Protein	Salt
	473	21g	6g	57g	5g	13g	16g	2.5g

INGREDIENTS

- 1 ⅓ cups / 200g green beans, trimmed and halved
- 2 tbsp olive oil
- 14 oz / 400g can chickpeas, rinsed
- 1 garlic clove, chopped
- ½ cup / 30g sundried tomatoes
- 1 whole roasted red pepper from jar
- ½ tbsp red wine vinegar
- ⅓ cup / 50g feta cheese

METHOD

01/ Heat oven to 400F (200C). Add beans to baking tray, season and drizzle over half of the oil. Roast for 10 minutes until lightly charred. Tip into a bowl with the chickpeas

02/ In a food processor, whizz together the garlic, tomatoes, peppers, vinegar and oil. Season, stir into the beans with the feta and serve.

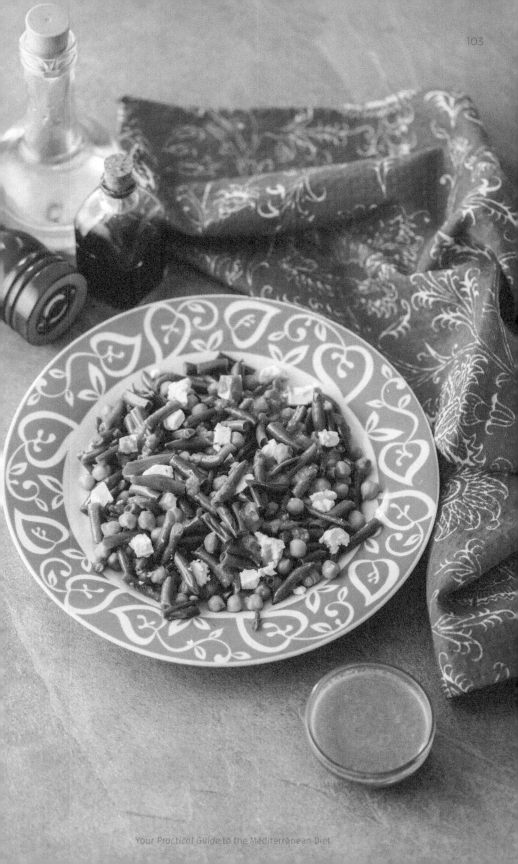

Spicy Quinoa & Almond Salad

SUITABLE
Quick

PREP TIME
10 mins

COOK TIME
15 mins

SERVES
4

Nutrition (per serving)	Kcal	Fat	Sat Fat	Carb	Sugar	Fibre	Protein	Salt
	450	20g	5g	51g	2g	7g	17g	0.7g

INGREDIENTS

1 tbsp olive oil

1 tsp ground cilantro

½ tsp turmeric

1 ½ cups / 300g quinoa, rinsed

½ cup / 50g toasted flaked almonds

⅔ cup / 100g feta cheese, crumbled

handful of parsley, chopped

juice ½ lemon

METHOD

01/ Heat the oil in a large pan. Add the spices, then fry for a minute. Add the quinoa and fry for a further minute. Stir in 600ml of boiling water, then gently simmer for 10-15 minutes until the water has evaporated. Let the quinoa cool slightly, then add other ingredients. Serve warm or cold.

Notes:

Try adding some cherry tomatoes, black olives or avocado to add some extra flavor. Keeps for a few days, so it's great if you want to batch-cook lunches.

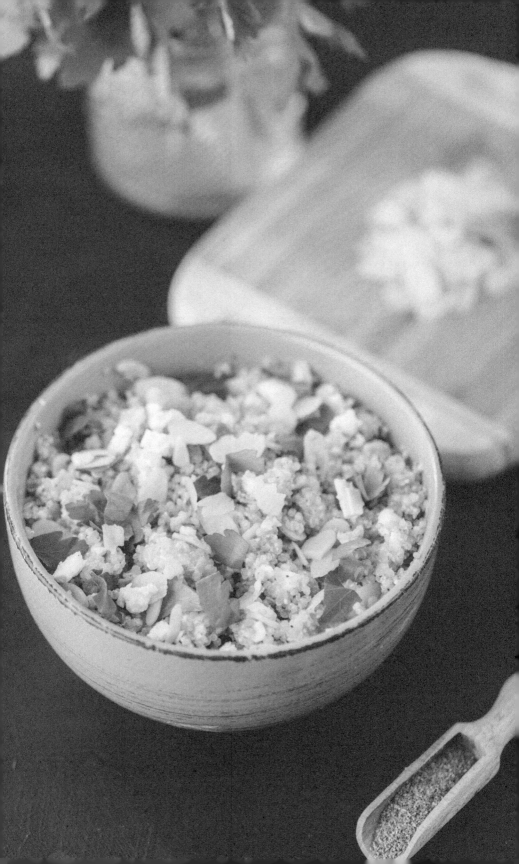

Chickpea, Pepper & Spiced Bulgur Wheat

SUITABLE
Vegan/Quick

PREP TIME
10 mins

COOK TIME
15 mins

SERVES
2

Nutrition (per serving)	Kcal	Fat	Sat Fat	Carb	Sugar	Fibre	Protein	Salt
	300	9g	2g	43g	4g	10g	9g	1.5g

INGREDIENTS

1 cup 200g bulgur wheat

½ cup / 25ml hot vegetable stock

1 tsp ground cumin

1 tsp ground cinnamon

zest and juice ½ lemon

1 tbsp olive oil

½ red onion, finely sliced

7 oz / 200g can chickpeas, drained

⅔ / 100g jar roasted pepper, torn

bunch of cilantro, leaves only

METHOD

01/ In a large bowl, cover bulgur wheat with stock. Cover with cling film and microwave on high for 4 minutes. Set aside for 5 minutes, covered. Make a dressing with cumin, cinnamon, lemon zest, juice and olive oil, then season. Add the onion, chickpeas, peppers, cilantro and cooked bulgur wheat. Serve warm or cold.

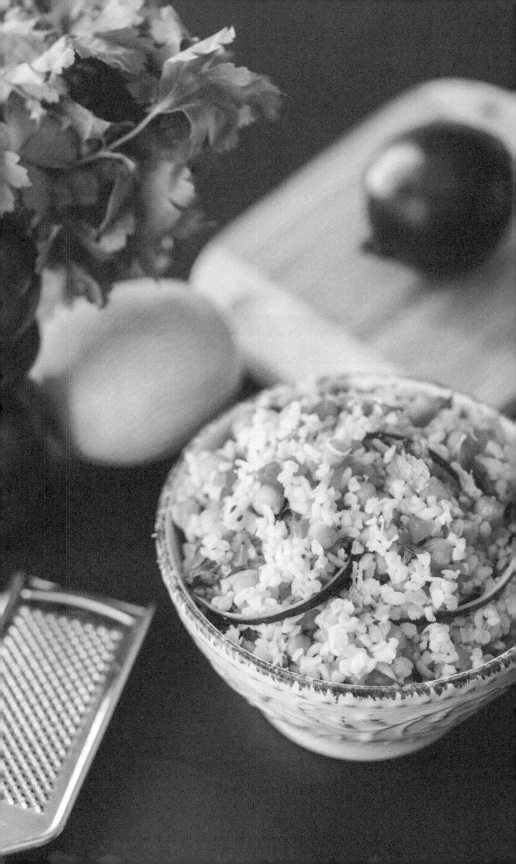

Roast Carrot & Bean Salad with Feta

SUITABLE
/

PREP TIME
10 mins

COOK TIME
30 mins

SERVES
2

Nutrition (per serving)	Kcal	Fat	Sat Fat	Carb	Sugar	Fibre	Protein	Salt
	437	26g	9g	41g	16g	13g	14g	2.0g

INGREDIENTS

2 cups / 500g baby carrots

2 tbsp olive oil

¾ cup / 90g green beans, halved

7 oz / 200g can cannellini beans, drained and rinsed

½ red onion, halved and sliced

⅔ cup / 100g feta cheese

small bunch mint, torn

METHOD

01/ Heat oven to 425F (220C). Put the carrots into a large roasting tin, add 1 tbsp oil, then season well. Roast for about 30 minutes until golden, turning halfway.

02/ Meanwhile, cook the green beans in boiling water for 2 minutes. Drain, cool under cold running water, then drain again. Mix together the green beans, cannellini, remaining oil, onion and feta, then season. Add the carrots and mint before serving.

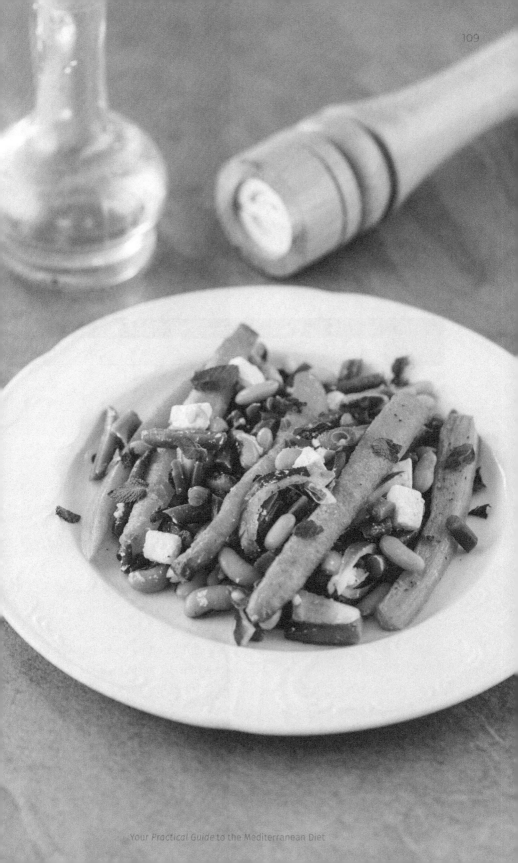

Spicy Mediterranean Beet Salad

SUITABLE

/

PREP TIME

10 mins

COOK TIME

30 mins

SERVES

2

Nutrition (per serving)	Kcal	Fat	Sat Fat	Carb	Sugar	Fibre	Protein	Salt
	548	20g	4g	58g	6g	11g	23g	1.7g

INGREDIENTS

- 8 raw baby beetroots, or 4 medium, scrubbed
- ½ tbsp za'atar
- ½ tbsp sumac
- ½ tbsp ground cumin
- 14 oz / 400g can chickpeas, drained and rinsed
- 2 tbsp olive oil
- ½ tsp lemon zest
- ½ tsp lemon juice
- ⅘ cup / 200g Greek yogurt
- 1 tbsp harissa paste
- 1 tsp crushed red chilli flakes
- mint leaves, chopped, to serve

METHOD

01/ Heat oven to 425F (220C). Halve or quarter beetroots depending on size. Mix spices together. On a large baking tray, mix chickpeas and beetroot with the oil. Season with salt & sprinkle over the spices. Mix again. Roast for 30 minutes.

02/ While the vegetables are cooking, mix the lemon zest and juice with the yogurt. Swirl the harissa through and spread into a bowl. Top with the beetroot & chickpeas, and sprinkle with the chilli flakes & mint.

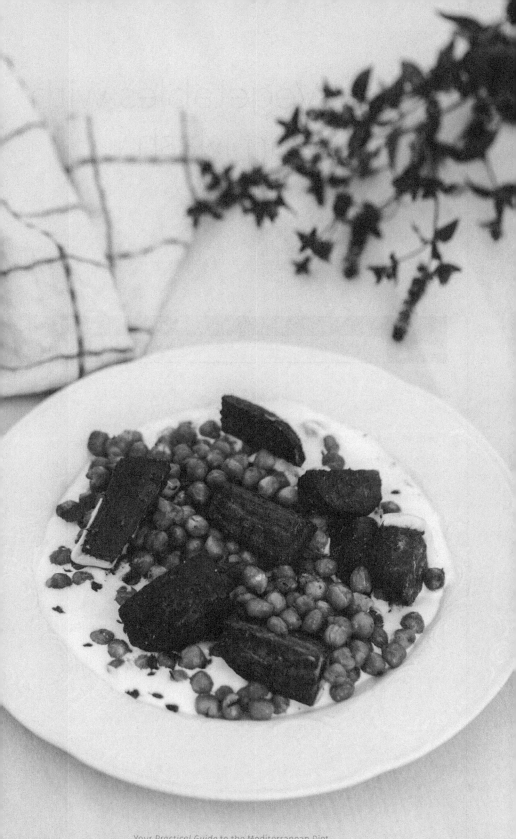

Grilled Vegetables with Bean Mash

SUITABLE	**PREP TIME**	**COOK TIME**	**SERVES**
Vegan	15 mins	25 mins	2

Nutrition (per serving)	Kcal	Fat	Sat Fat	Carb	Sugar	Fibre	Protein	Salt
	314	16g	2g	33g	9g	11g	19g	0.1g

INGREDIENTS

1 pepper, deseeded & quartered

1 eggplant / aubergine, sliced lengthways

2 zucchini / courgettes, sliced lengthways

2 tbsp olive oil

For the mash

14 oz / 400g can haricot beans, rinsed

1 garlic clove, crushed

½ cup / 100ml vegetable stock

1 tbsp chopped cilantro

METHOD

01/ Heat the grill. Arrange the vegetables over a grill pan & brush lightly with oil. Grill until lightly browned, turn them over, brush again with oil, then grill until tender.

02/ Meanwhile, put the beans in a pan with garlic and stock. Bring to a boil, then simmer, uncovered, for 10 minutes. Mash roughly with a potato masher. Divide the vegetables and mash between 2 plates, drizzle over oil & sprinkle with black pepper & cilantro.

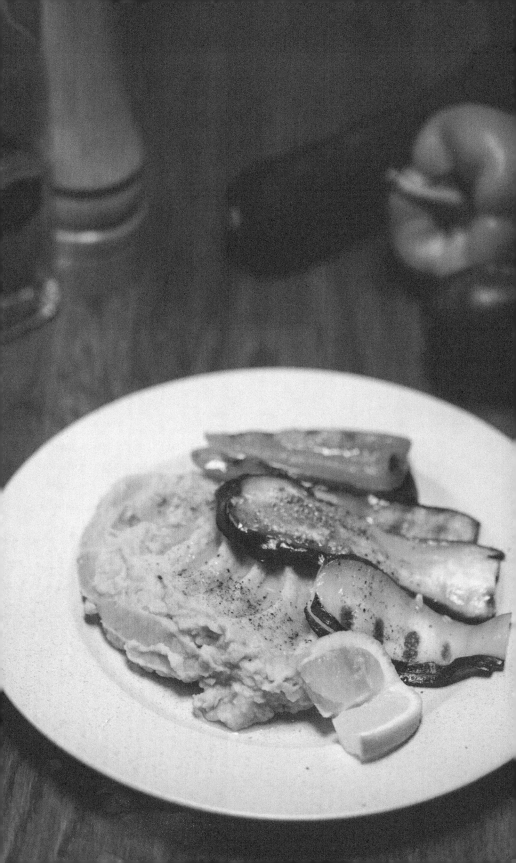

Grilled Eggplant Slices with Hummus

SUITABLE

Vegan/Quick

PREP TIME

10 mins

COOK TIME

15 mins

SERVES

2

Nutrition (per serving)	Kcal	Fat	Sat Fat	Carb	Sugar	Fibre	Protein	Salt
	552	37g	4g	49g	10g	17g	17g	1.4g

INGREDIENTS

1 eggplant / aubergine, sliced lengthways

2 tbsp olive oil

2 slices brown bread

⅗ cup / 150g hummus

½ cup / 50g walnut, toasted

1 ½ cups / 40g parsley, leaves chopped

⅔ cup / 100g cherry tomatoes, quartered

juice ½ lemon

METHOD

01 / Lay eggplant on baking sheet. Add olive oil, then season. Grill for 15 minutes, turning twice until cooked through. Whizz bread into crumbs.

02 / Spread hummus on eggplant slices. Tip breadcrumbs onto a plate, then press the hummus side of the eggplant into the crumbs to coat. Grill again, crumbside up, for 3 minutes. until golden.

03 / Add walnuts, parsley & tomatoes in a bowl, season, then add lemon juice. Serve with salad.

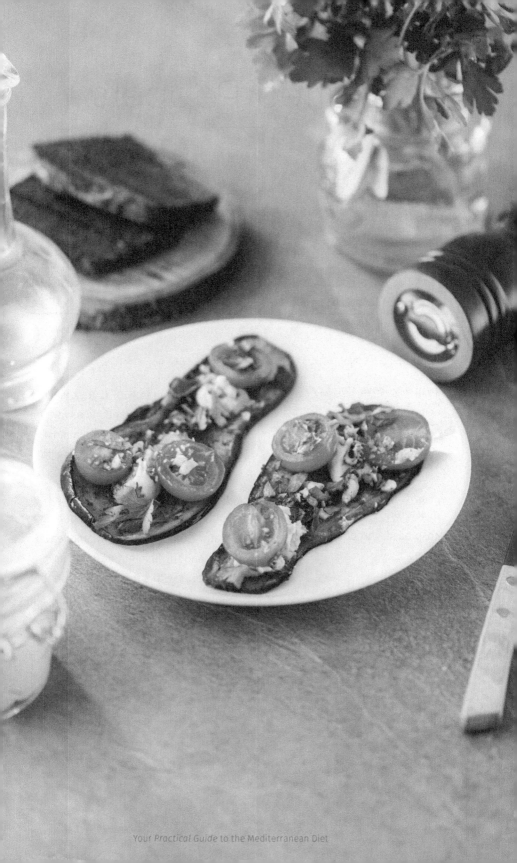

Stuffed Peppers

SUITABLE

/

PREP TIME

15 mins

COOK TIME

25 mins

SERVES

2

Nutrition (per serving)	Kcal	Fat	Sat Fat	Carb	Sugar	Fibre	Protein	Salt
	642	29g	8g	62g	4g	6g	23g	1.7g

INGREDIENTS

4 peppers *(leave stalks on)*

¾ cup / 140g couscous

½ cup / 50g walnuts, toasted

handful black olives, chopped

⅔ cup / 100g feta cheese, crumbled

⅔ cup / 100g cherry tomatoes, quartered

4 tbsp basil, shredded

METHOD

01/ Heat oven to 400F (200C). Place peppers on a plate and microwave on medium for 5 minutes, until almost soft. Place on a baking tray, cutside up.

02/ Meanwhile, place the couscous in a bowl and cover with 125ml boiling water. Stir, cover the bowl and leave to stand for 10 minutes. Break up couscous with a fork, then mix in the nuts, olives, feta, tomatoes and basil. Pile the couscous stuffing into the pepper halves & bake for 10 minutes.

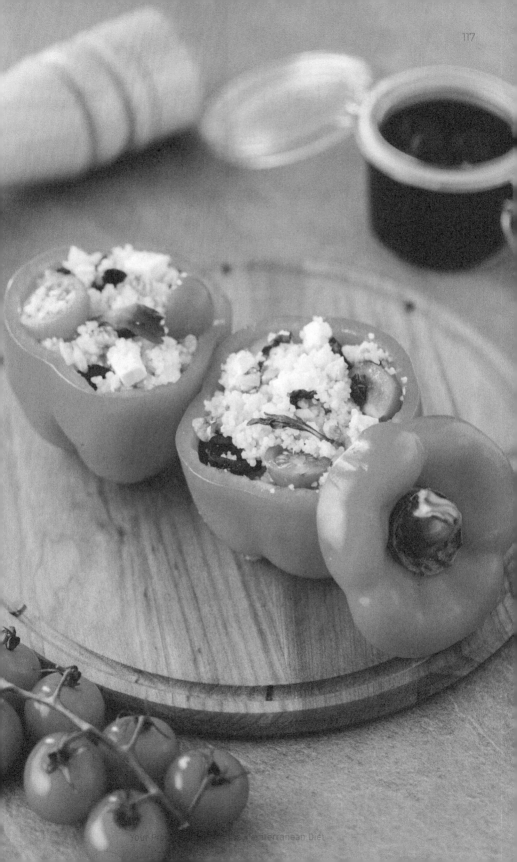

Eggplant Lentil Bake

SUITABLE	PREP TIME	COOK TIME	SERVES
/	15 mins	45 mins	2

Nutrition (per serving)	Kcal	Fat	Sat Fat	Carb	Sugar	Fibre	Protein	Salt
	444	20g	6g	52g	12g	19g	17g	0.7g

INGREDIENTS

1 eggplant / aubergine, sliced lengthways

2 tbsp olive oil

⅓ cup / 70g lentils

2 onions, finely chopped

2 garlic cloves, finely chopped

¾ cup / 150g cooked butternut squash

7 oz / 200g can chopped tomatoes

½ small pack basil leaves

⅓ cup / 60g feta

METHOD

01/ Heat oven to 425F (220C). Add oil to each eggplant side. Lay on baking sheets, season and bake for 15-20 minutes, turning once. Cook lentils following pack instructions.

02/ Heat oil in frying pan. Add onions and garlic and cook until soft. Add squash & tomatoes, plus ½ can of water. Simmer for 10-15 minutes until the sauce thickens. Stir in lentils, basil & seasoning.

03/ Spoon layer of lentils into baking dish, then eggplant slices and repeat. Scatter feta and bake for 15 more minutes until cheese is golden.

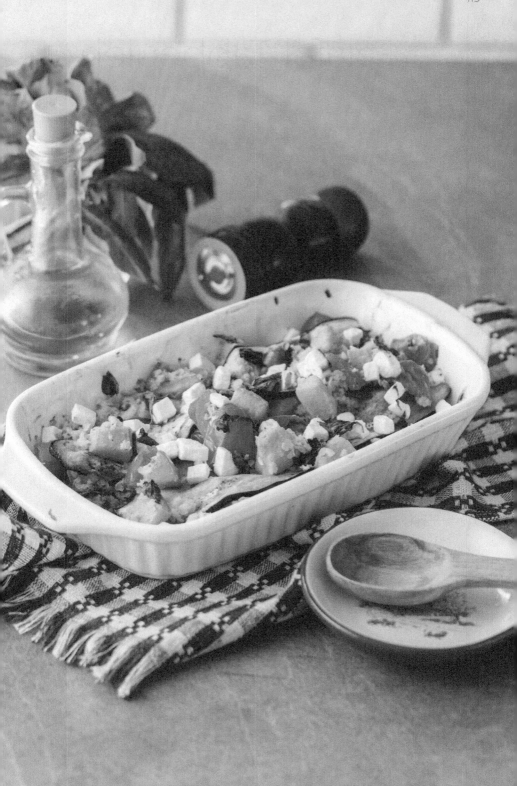

Falafel Tabbouleh

SUITABLE

Quick

PREP TIME

5 mins

COOK TIME

15 mins

SERVES

2

Nutrition (per serving)	Kcal	Fat	Sat Fat	Carb	Sugar	Fibre	Protein	Salt
	653	36g	4g	67g	4g	6g	17g	1.4g

INGREDIENTS

8 ready-made falafel

½ cup / 100g couscous

1 large lemon, zest and juice

3 tbsp olive oil

bunch spring onions, finely sliced

1 cucumber, halved and sliced

small bunch mint, leaves chopped

bunch parsley, leaves roughly chopped

4 tbsp Greek yogurt

METHOD

01/ Cook the falafels according to pack instructions and boil the kettle. Tip the couscous into a large bowl, pour over 300ml boiling water, cover, then leave to stand for 5 minutes until all of the water is absorbed.

02/ Fluff up the couscous with a fork, then stir through the lemon zest, juice from the lemon, olive oil, spring onions, cucumber, mint and three-quarters of the parsley with plenty of seasoning. Tip onto a large platter.

03/ Mix the remaining lemon juice and parsley into the yogurt, then spoon into a small bowl. Scatter the hot falafel over the couscous salad and serve the yogurt sauce alongside.

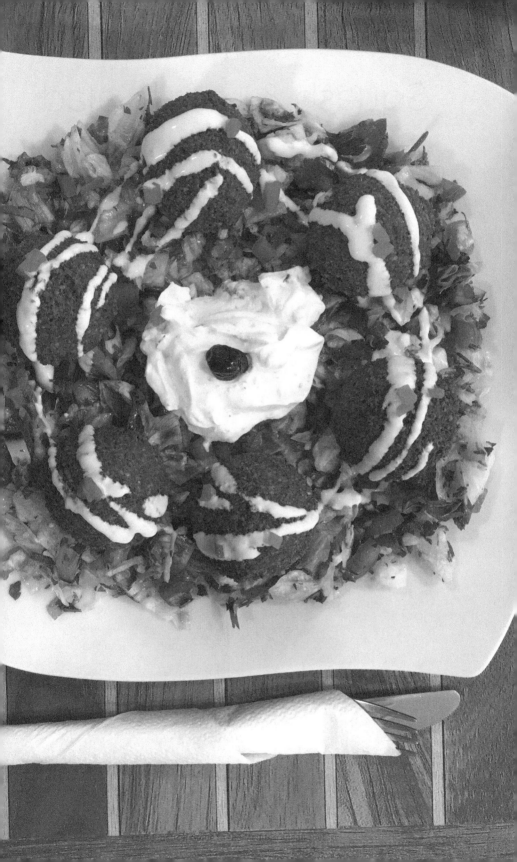

Squash & Lentil Salad

SUITABLE

/

PREP TIME

10 mins

COOK TIME

30 mins

SERVES

2

Nutrition (per serving)	Kcal	Fat	Sat Fat	Carb	Sugar	Fibre	Protein	Salt
	409	14g	3g	58g	9g	13g	17g	1.1g

INGREDIENTS

2 ½ cups / 500g butternut squash, diced

1 tbsp olive oil

1 garlic clove, crushed

1 tsp basil leaves

½ tbsp red wine vinegar

1 tsp wholegrain mustard

14 oz / 400g can lentils

½ red onion sliced

1 ⅔ cups / 50g spinach

½ cup / 75g cherry tomatoes, halved

⅙ cup / 20g feta cheese

1 tbsp mixed seeds

METHOD

01 / Heat oven to 400F (200C). On a baking tray, place butternut squash, olive oil, garlic clove, basil & seasoning. Roast for 25-30 minutes or until tender.

02 / Mix together vinegar, ½ tbsp olive oil, wholegrain mustard and 1-2 tbsp water. Drain the water from the puy lentils and add the red onion, spinach and tomatoes.

03 / Divide the lentils between plates. Top with the butternut squash, then crumble over feta cheese and sprinkle the mixed seeds.

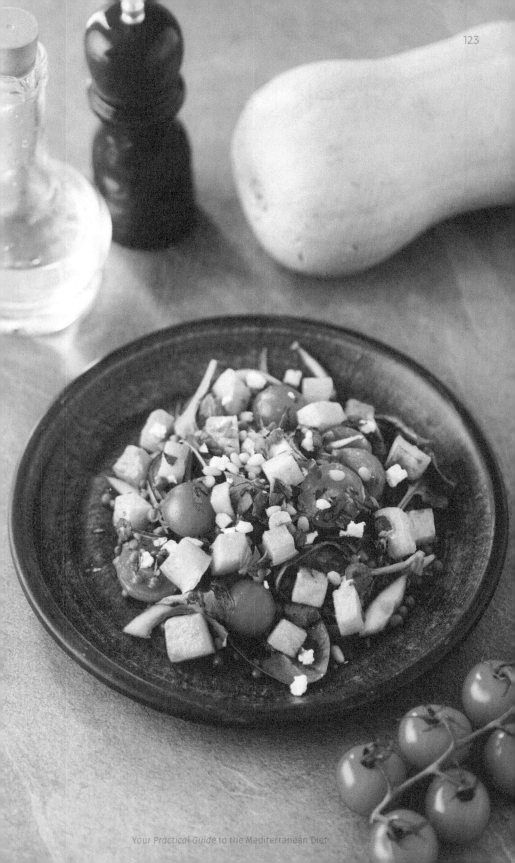

Greek Pasta Salad

SUITABLE

/

PREP TIME

5 mins

COOK TIME

35 mins

SERVES

4

Nutrition (per serving)	Kcal	Fat	Sat Fat	Carb	Sugar	Fibre	Protein	Salt
	554	26g	9g	64g	7g	9g	19g	0.3g

INGREDIENTS

1 ½ cups / 300g whole wheat fusilli/ farfalle/penne pasta

7-8 cups / 225g baby spinach

1 ½ cups / 250g cherry tomatoes, halved

½ cup / 100g black olives

1 ⅓ cups / 200g feta cheese

3 tbsp olive oil

METHOD

01/ Tip pasta into a pan of boiling salted water and boil for 10 minutes. Throw in the spinach, stir well and boil for another 2 minutes. Drain into a colander or sieve.

02/ Tip the tomatoes, olives and feta into a large bowl, add lots of black pepper and drizzle with the olive oil.

03/ Toss in the drained pasta and spinach and serve.

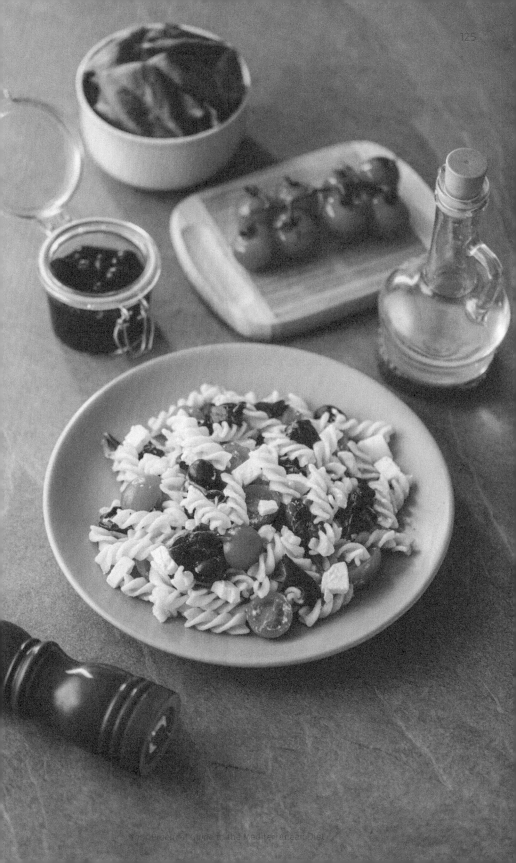

Carrot, Sweet Potato & Ginger Soup

SUITABLE	**PREP TIME**	**COOK TIME**	**SERVES**
Gluten Free	5 mins	20 mins	2

Nutrition (per serving)	Kcal	Fat	Sat Fat	Carb	Sugar	Fibre	Protein	Salt
	302	17g	2g	30g	9g	4g	6g	0.2g

INGREDIENTS

1 tsp olive oil

1 onion

1 thumb sized piece ginger root, grated

1 sweet potato

3 medium carrots

½ cup / 50g ground almonds

2 ½ cups / 600ml vegetable stock

Topping

2 tbsp Greek yogurt

2 tbsp pistachios, chopped

2 tbsp chopped dried apple rings

salt and pepper to season

METHOD

01/ Heat the oil in a saucepan and add the ginger and onion. Stir over a medium heat, cooking the onion and ginger for 3-4 minutes until softened. Add the rest of the ingredients and cover.

02/ Simmer for 15-20 minutes until all the ingredients are soft. Using a hand blender, carefully blend the soup until completely smooth.

03/ Serve between two bowls and add swirls of Greek yoghurt. Add plenty of black pepper and sprinkle on the nuts and apple pieces.

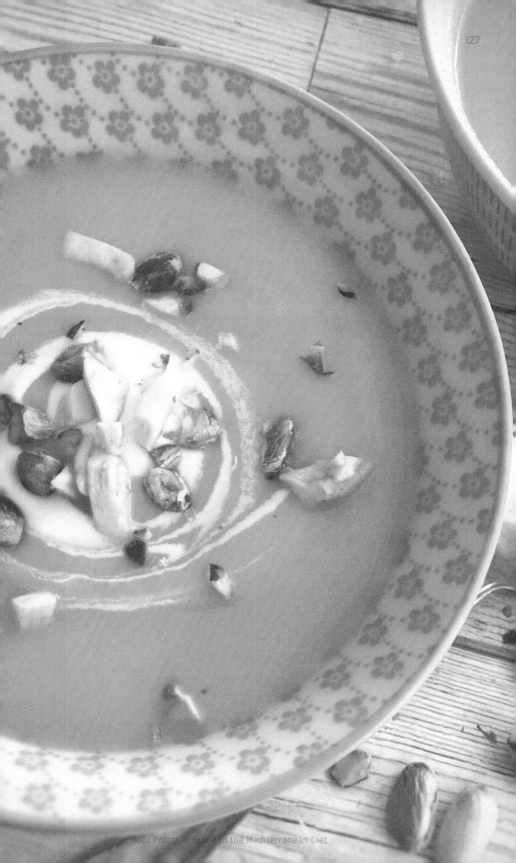

Spicy Tomato Baked Eggs

SUITABLE
Quick

PREP TIME
5 mins

COOK TIME
20 mins

SERVES
2

Nutrition (per serving)	Kcal	Fat	Sat Fat	Carb	Sugar	Fibre	Protein	Salt
	417	17g	4g	45g	7g	5g	19g	0.8g

INGREDIENTS

1 tbsp olive oil

2 red onions, chopped

1 red chilli, deseeded & chopped

1 garlic clove, sliced

small bunch cilantro, stalks and leaves chopped separately

2 x 14 oz / 2 x 400g can cherry tomatoes

4 eggs

brown bread, to serve

METHOD

01/ Heat the oil in a frying pan with a lid, then cook the onions, chilli, garlic and cilantro stalks for 5 minutes until soft. Stir in the tomatoes, then simmer for 8-10 minutes.

02/ Using the back of a large spoon, make 4 dips in the sauce, then crack an egg into each one. Put a lid on the pan, then cook over a low heat for 6-8 mins, until the eggs are done to your liking. Scatter with the cilantro leaves and serve with bread.

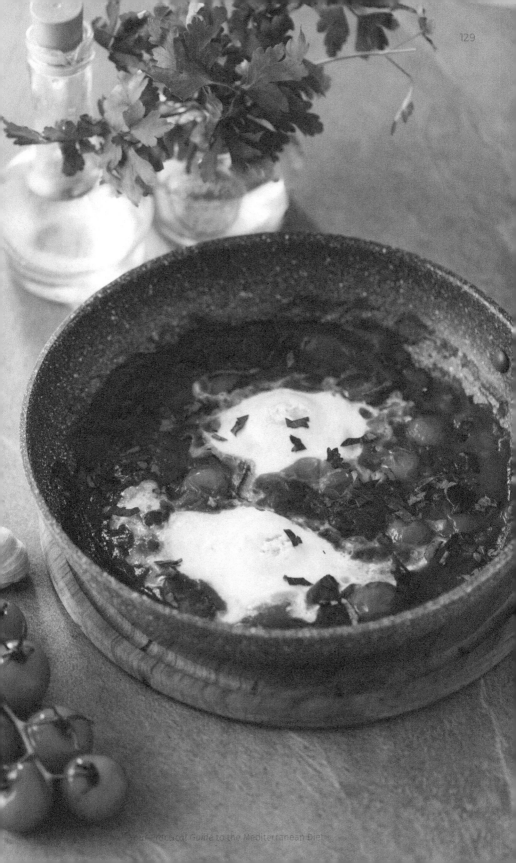

Maltese Garlic Beans & Herbs

———

SUITABLE
Vegan/Quick

PREP TIME
5 mins

COOK TIME
15 mins

SERVES
2

Nutrition (per serving)	Kcal	Fat	Sat Fat	Carb	Sugar	Fibre	Protein	Salt
	394	14g	2g	53g	12g	15g	16g	2.4g

INGREDIENTS

7-8 baby carrots

small eggplant wedge, cut into chunks

2 garlic cloves, crushed

1 tsp fennel seeds

2 tbsp rolled oats

2 tbsp extra virgin olive oil

1 tin butterbeans (*or other*)

2 tbsp black beans

I small leek, sliced

1 tsp salt

pea shoots, to serve

METHOD

01/ In a saucepan, heat the oil. Add the leek & stir for 3-4 minutes, until soft. Add the fennel & garlic. Over a low heat, let the garlic soften & the fennel release its flavor into the pan. Stir in the beans & rolled oats.

02/ Roast the vegetables with a little of the oil from the pan & add salt.

03/ When the vegetables are cooked, divide between plates. Place a serving of beans beside them & drizzle over any remaining oats & oil from the pan. Serve with pea shoots.

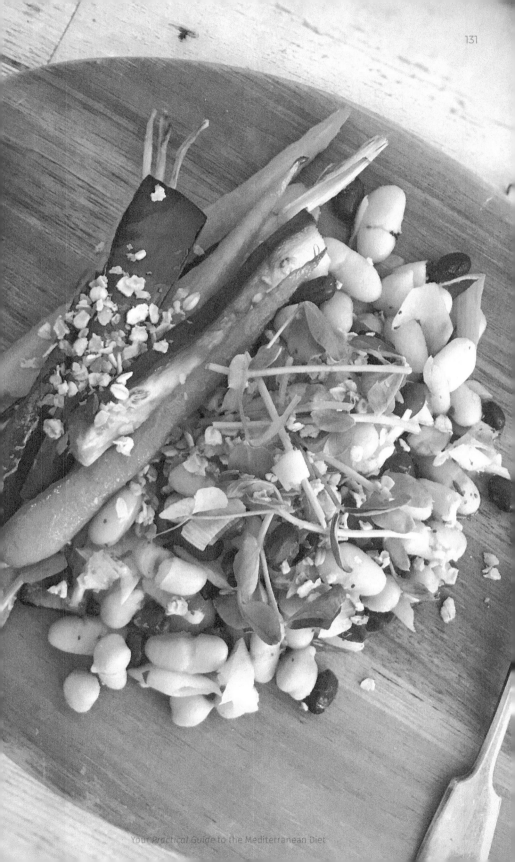

Buddha Bowl with Spiced Vegetables

SUITABLE	**PREP TIME**	**COOK TIME**	**SERVES**
Vegan/Quick	5 mins	5 mins	2

Nutrition (per serving)	Kcal	Fat	Sat Fat	Carb	Sugar	Fibre	Protein	Salt
	358	11g	2g	48g	10g	10g	15g	1.4g

INGREDIENTS

1 small beetroot, raw, peeled, grated

½ tin of chickpeas

1 tsp olive oil

½ onion, diced

½ tsp ground cumin

½ tsp ground sumac

1 zucchini / courgette, sliced

1 small carrot, sliced

1/2 green pepper, sliced

7 oz / 200g tin chopped tomatoes

1 ½ cups / 250g pouch quinoa

1 tbsp soy yoghurt, plus ½ tsp extra sumac to dust on top

2 tbsp pumpkin seeds

METHOD

01/ In a saucepan, heat the oil. Add the onion and stir for 3-4 minutes, until soft. Add the carrot and cook for a further 4-5 minutes. Add the tomatoes, spices, zucchini, pepper and salt and cook for a further 5 minutes until softened. Leave to cool. You could do this in advance and just "assemble" the bowl when you are ready to eat.

02/ Place strips of each ingredient into two bowls. Divide the yoghurt between them and sprinkle over the extra sumac. Scatter over the pumpkin seeds and serve.

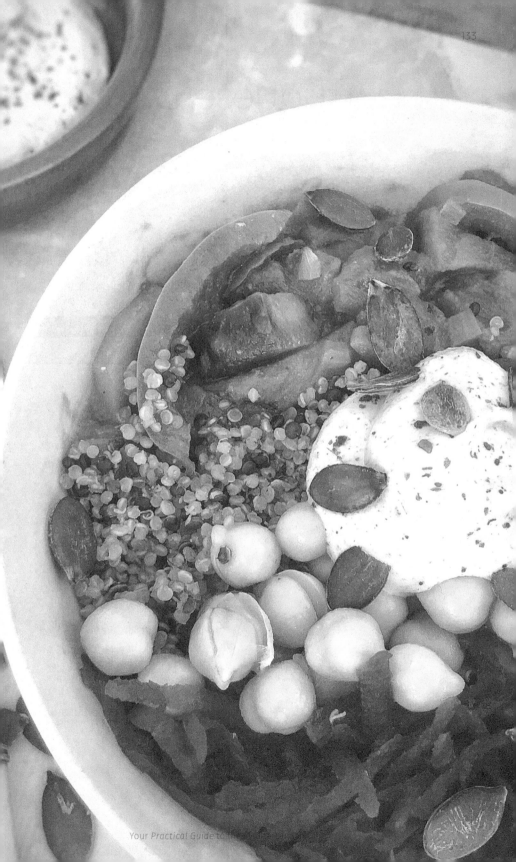

Portuguese Baked Eggs

SUITABLE

/

PREP TIME

5 mins

COOK TIME

30 mins

SERVES

2

Nutrition (per serving)	Kcal	Fat	Sat Fat	Carb	Sugar	Fibre	Protein	Salt
	264	10g	3g	25g	13g	6g	16g	2g

INGREDIENTS

4 eggs

1 tsp olive oil

1 onion, finely chopped

1 garlic clove, crushed

1 small eggplant / aubergine

1 green bell pepper

1 medium carrot sliced

1 tin of chopped Tomatoes

1 tsp dried oregano

1 tsp honey

1 tp salt

METHOD

01/ In a saucepan, heat the oil. Add onion & garlic & stir for 3-4 minutes, until soft. Add vegetables & cook for 4-5 minutes until soft. Add tomatoes, oregano, salt & honey & cook for 10 minutes until sauce thickens.

02/ Pre-heat the oven to 400F (200C) & grease a small casserole dish. Tip the tomato & vegetable sauce into the bottom of the dish. Make 4 "dents" in the sauce with a back of a spoon & crack the eggs into each.

03/ Bake in the oven for 7-8 minutes, until the eggs are cooked but still runny in the middle.

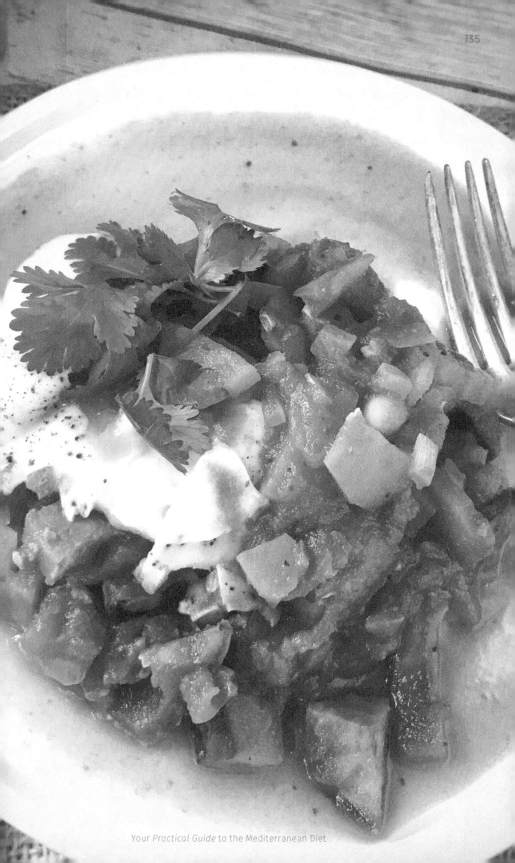

Sweet Potato and Peppers M'hanacha

SUITABLE
Vegan

PREP TIME
10 mins

COOK TIME
40 mins

SERVES
2

Nutrition (per serving)	Kcal	Fat	Sat Fat	Carb	Sugar	Fibre	Protein	Salt
	388	13g	2g	57g	12g	8g	11g	2g

INGREDIENTS

6 sheets filo pastry

1 tbsp olive oil

1 tbsp flaked almonds

For the Filling

1 tsp olive oil

1 red onion, chopped finely

1 garlic clove, crushed

½ tsp ground cumin

1 tsp ground cilantro

1 sweet potato, cut into cubes

1 red bell pepper, sliced

½ red chilli, seeds removed, diced

1 handful of shredded kale

METHOD

01/ In a saucepan, heat oil. Add onion & stir for 3-4 minutes. Add sweet potato, pepper, chilli & spices & stir over a medium heat for 10 minutes until potatoes are tender. Add kale & stir for a further 4 minutes until wilted. Cool mixture.

02/ Pre-heat the oven to 400F (200C) and grease a baking sheet. Lay the filo sheets (reserve half a sheet) on baking tray. Brush oil on pastry. Add filling onto pastry & create a thin sausage. Wrap short edges over vegetables to seal ends & roll the pastry to create a long sausage shape. Use remaining pastry & oil to cover any holes. Sprinkle almonds & bake for 25 minutes.

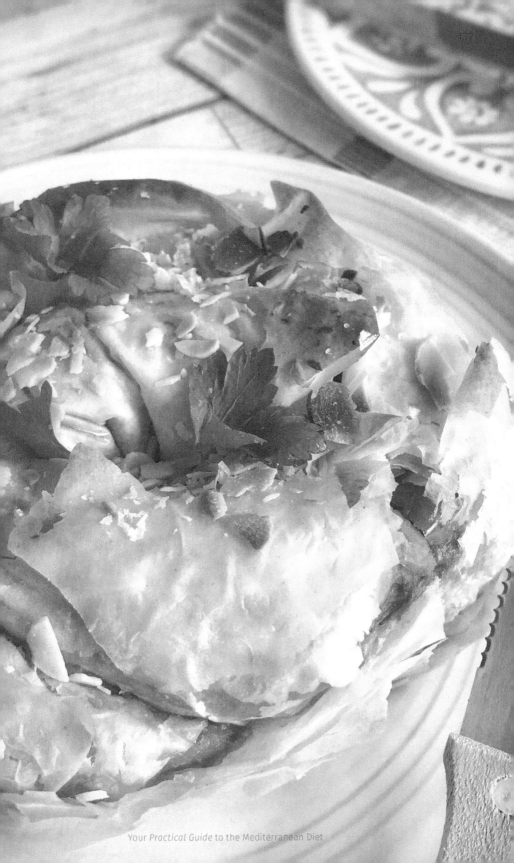

Lentil & Fennel Salad

SUITABLE
Vegan/Quick

PREP TIME
10 mins

COOK TIME
10 mins

SERVES
2

Nutrition (per serving)	Kcal	Fat	Sat Fat	Carb	Sugar	Fibre	Protein	Salt
	415	20g	1g	40g	9g	8g	19g	2.8g

INGREDIENTS

¼ cup / 250g ready cooked puy lentils

3 tsp olive oil

2 tsp balsamic vinegar

1 lemon, zest only

1 fennel bulb, sliced

9-10 baby plum tomatoes, sliced

7-8 black olives, sliced

salt

parsley & brown bread, to serve

METHOD

01/ Pre-heat the oven to 400F (200C) and grease a baking tray. Place the fennel slices on the tray and drizzle with 1 tsp of the oil and a little sea salt. Roast for 10 minutes until soft and a little crisp around the edges.

02/ Mix the lentils with the olives and tomatoes and divide between two plates. Mix the lemon juice with the oil and balsamic vinegar. Place the fennel on top of the lentils and drizzle over the dressing.

03/ Serve with bread & fresh parsley.

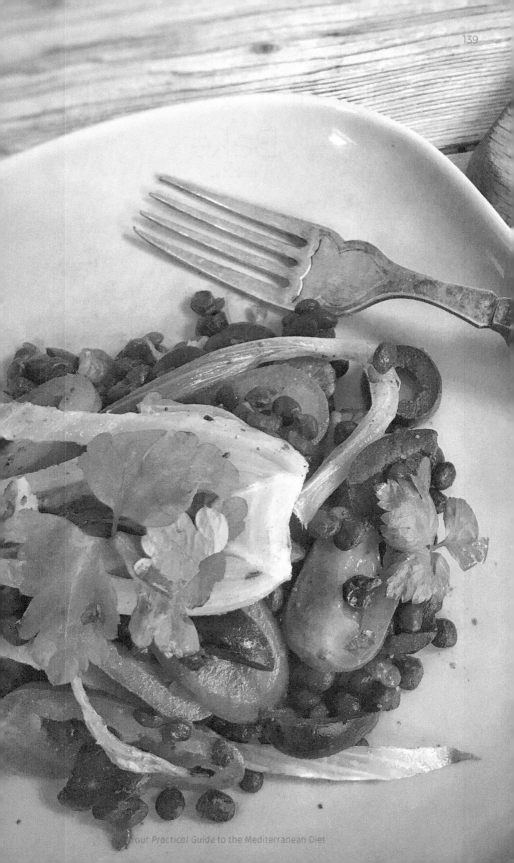

Zucchini & Gnocchi Bake

SUITABLE
Vegan/Quick

PREP TIME
5 mins

COOK TIME
15 mins

SERVES
2

Nutrition (per serving)	Kcal	Fat	Sat Fat	Carb	Sugar	Fibre	Protein	Salt
	355	10g	1g	58g	6g	10g	18g	0.9g

INGREDIENTS

1 tsp olive oil

1 red onion, halved and sliced

½ tin chickpeas

1 ¼ cups / 250g gnocchi

1 small zucchini / courgette, sliced

1 lemon, zest only

1 tsp dried oregano

1 tsp salt

1 large handful of kale

1 tsp extra-virgin olive oil

METHOD

01/ In a saucepan, heat the oil. Add the onion and stir for 3-4 minutes, until soft. Add the gnocchi, zucchini, chickpeas & lemon zest to the pan, with a splash of water. Heat over a medium heat until the gnocchi has swollen and browned a little and heated through. Add the kale and stir until it begins to wilt.

02/ Just before serving, stir through the extra virgin olive oil & herbs. Serve immediately.

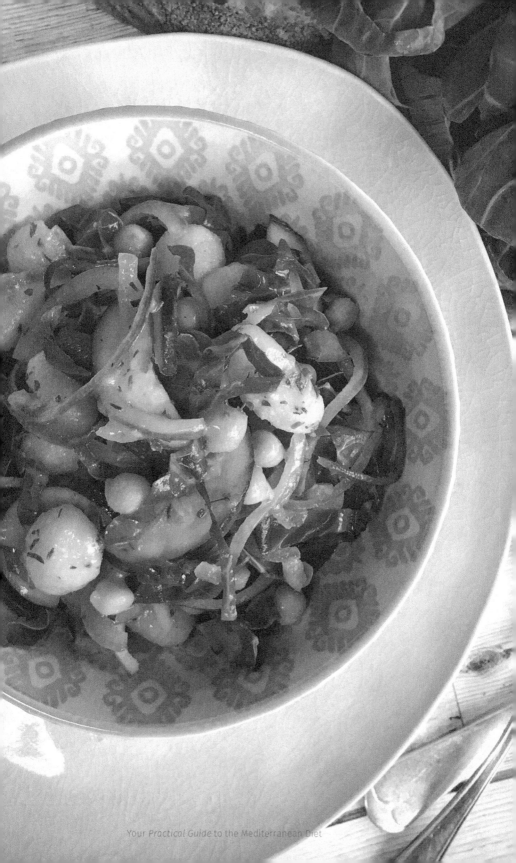

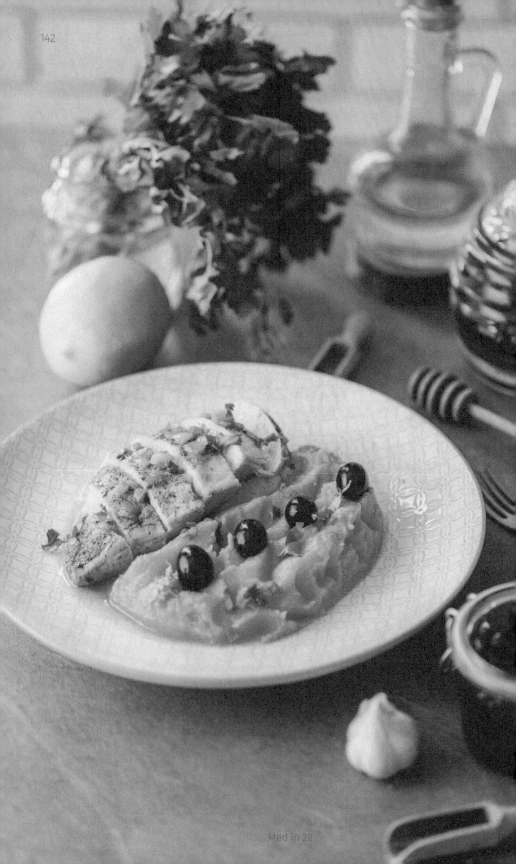

Poultry

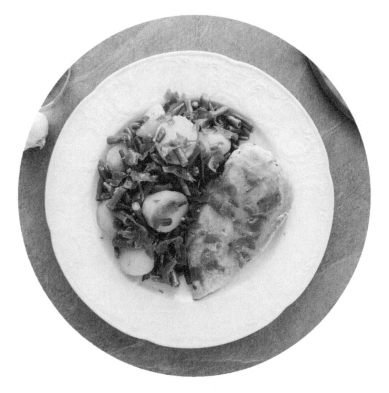

Pollo Español Hornear

SUITABLE
High Protein

PREP TIME
10 mins

COOK TIME
35 mins

SERVES
2

Nutrition (per serving)	Kcal	Fat	Sat Fat	Carb	Sugar	Fibre	Protein	Salt
	508	15g	4g	51g	6g	6g	40g	0.9g

INGREDIENTS

1 tbsp harissa paste

1 tbsp red wine vinegar

2 chicken breasts

1 red onion, cut into quarters

1 pepper, sliced

⅓ cup / 50g feta cheese

⅙ cup / 25g almonds, toasted

½ cup / 100g couscous, cooked following pack instructions, to serve

METHOD

01 / Heat oven to 400F (200C). In a large bowl, mix the harissa paste and the red wine vinegar, then add the chicken, pepper and onions. Spread the mixture out in a large roasting tin and roast for 35 minutes, turning at least once.

02 / In the final 10 minutes, add the peppers and feta, then sprinkle with the almonds just before the end of the cooking time. Serve with the pan juices and couscous.

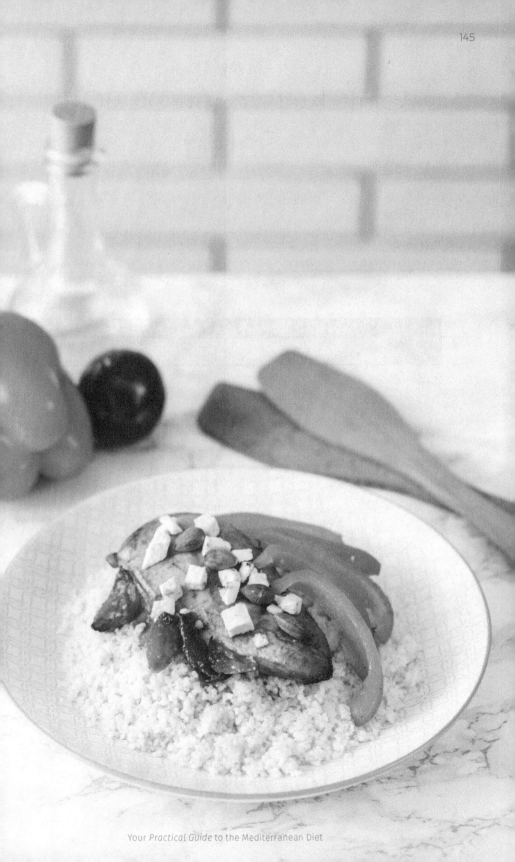

Chicken & Avocado Salad

SUITABLE
Quick

PREP TIME
10 mins

COOK TIME
10 mins

SERVES
2

Nutrition (per serving)	Kcal	Fat	Sat Fat	Carb	Sugar	Fibre	Protein	Salt
	396	26g	5g	15g	4g	9g	31g	0.2g

INGREDIENTS

2 chicken breast

2 tsp olive oil *(1 for the salad)*

2 tsp smoked paprika

For the salad

1 small avocado, diced

½ tsp red wine vinegar

½ tbsp parsley, chopped

⅘ cup / 120g tomatoes, chopped

half small red onion, thinly sliced

METHOD

01/ Heat grill to medium. Rub the chicken with 1 tsp of the olive oil and the paprika. Cook for 4-5 minutes each side until lightly charred and cooked through.

02/ Mix the salad ingredients together, season and add the rest of the oil. Thickly slice the chicken and serve with the salad.

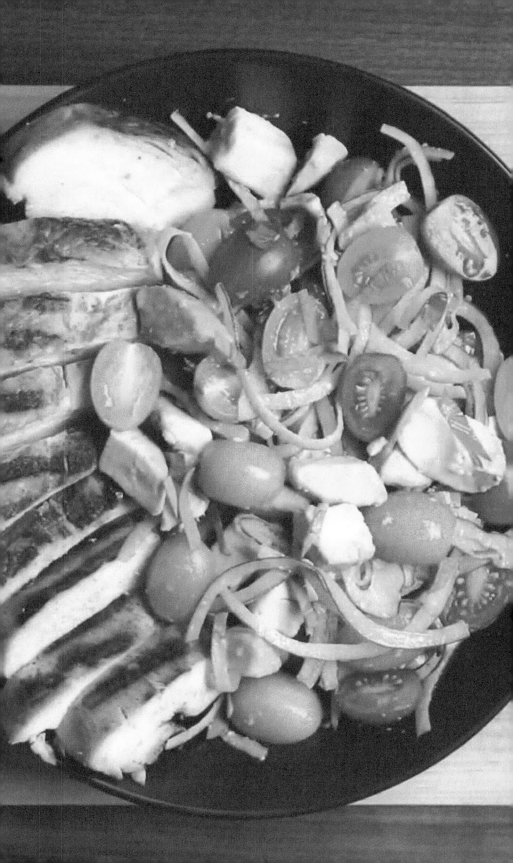

Citrus Chicken & Couscous

SUITABLE

Quick

PREP TIME

20 mins

COOK TIME

10 mins

SERVES

2

Nutrition (per serving)	Kcal	Fat	Sat Fat	Carb	Sugar	Fibre	Protein	Salt
	468	17g	1g	44g	3g	5g	36g	1.4g

INGREDIENTS

2 chicken breast

juice 1 lemon

1 tbsp olive oil

½ tsp dried chilli flakes

2 garlic cloves, crushed

For the couscous

½ cup / 100g couscous

¼ cup / 40g sultanas

½ cup / 125ml hot vegetable stock

¼ cup / 40g pitted black olives

7 oz / 200g can chickpeas, drained

1 tbsp parsley, chopped

METHOD

01/ Butterfly chicken breasts by cutting through the thickest part, stopping 1cm before the edge, then opening it out. Whisk together lemon juice, olive oil, chilli flakes & garlic. Pour half over the chicken and marinate for 15 minutes.

02/ Meanwhile, put the couscous & sultanas in a bowl, then pour over the stock. Cover the bowl with cling film & leave for 5 minutes.

03/ Heat a frying pan, remove the chicken from the marinade and cook for 4 minutes on each side until cooked through. Fluff up the couscous with a fork & stir in the olives, chickpeas, parsley & other half of marinade. Season & serve.

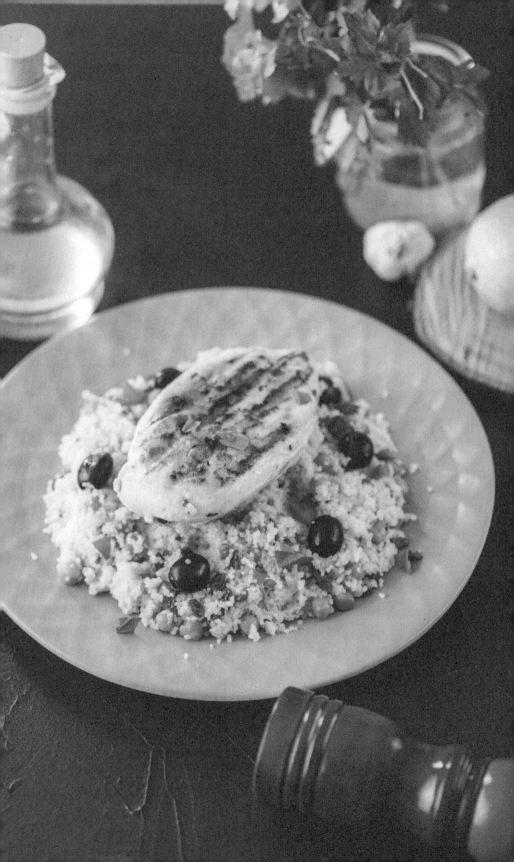

Chicken & Peach Fusion

SUITABLE
Quick

PREP TIME
10 mins

COOK TIME
15 mins

SERVES
2

Nutrition (per serving)	Kcal	Fat	Sat Fat	Carb	Sugar	Fibre	Protein	Salt
	384	22g	6g	20g	19g	3g	26g	0.8g

INGREDIENTS

1 ½ cups / 200g chicken breast

2 tbsp olive oil

2 ripe peaches, stoned and cut into quarters

2 tsp red wine vinegar

½ tbsp clear honey

½ red chilli, finely chopped

½ cup / 55g bag herb salad

⅓ cup / 50g feta cheese, crumbled

broccoli/green beans to serve (optional)

METHOD

01/ Heat a frying pan. Place the chicken in ½ tbsp of oil, and season. Cook for 3-4 minutes on each side until cooked through. Add to a plate.

02/ Place peach slices in ½ tbsp oil with black pepper. Grill for 1-2 minutes each side.

03/ Mix the remaining olive oil, vinegar, honey and chilli. Toss with the salad leaves. Arrange the chicken with the peach slices on top and scatter with feta before serving.

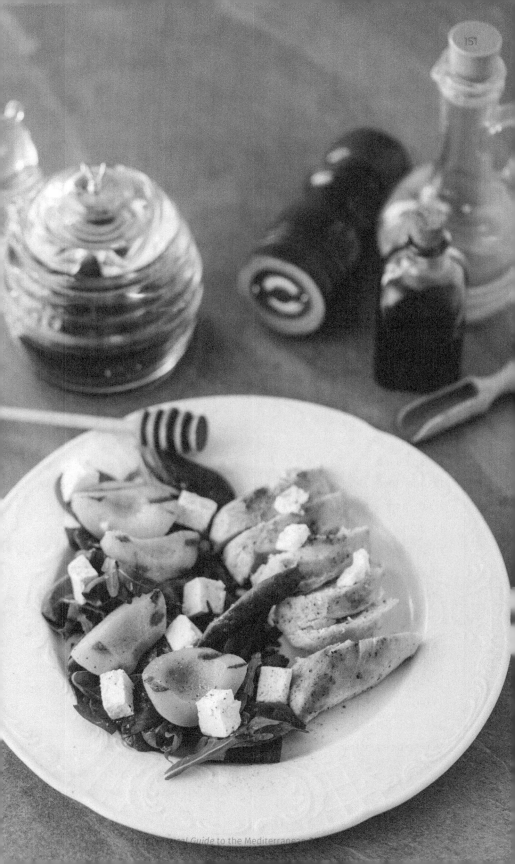

Baked Chicken Tapenade Salad Bowl

SUITABLE

Quick

PREP TIME

5 mins

COOK TIME

20 mins

SERVES

2

Nutrition (per serving)	Kcal	Fat	Sat Fat	Carb	Sugar	Fibre	Protein	Salt
	383	20g	3g	22g	5g	6g	32g	1.5g

INGREDIENTS

Topping

2 tbsp olives

1 garlic clove

2-3 tbsp olive oil

1 lemon, zest and juice

small bunch parsley

small sprig rosemary

salt

2 chicken breasts

7 oz / ½ tin cannellini beans

½ red pepper, thinly sliced

½ red onion, thinly sliced

3 ⅓ cups / 100g baby spinach

½ tbsp balsamic vinegar

METHOD

01/ Pre-heat the oven to 400F (200C) & grease or line a baking sheet or tray. Flatten chicken breasts between 2 sheets of cling film, until 1cm thick. Place onto baking tray.

02/ With a food processor or stick blender, whizz up garlic, oil, olives, lemon juice, zest & herbs to make a paste. Spread over chicken. Place chicken into the oven to bake for 16-18 minutes, until coloured on top & cooked. Leave to rest whilst making the salad and then slice into 2 pieces.

03/ Drain beans & rinse. In a bowl, mix the beans, onion, pepper, parsley, lemon juice, zest, oil & seasoning. Serve bean salad on plates, add spinach leaves, chicken & vinegar.

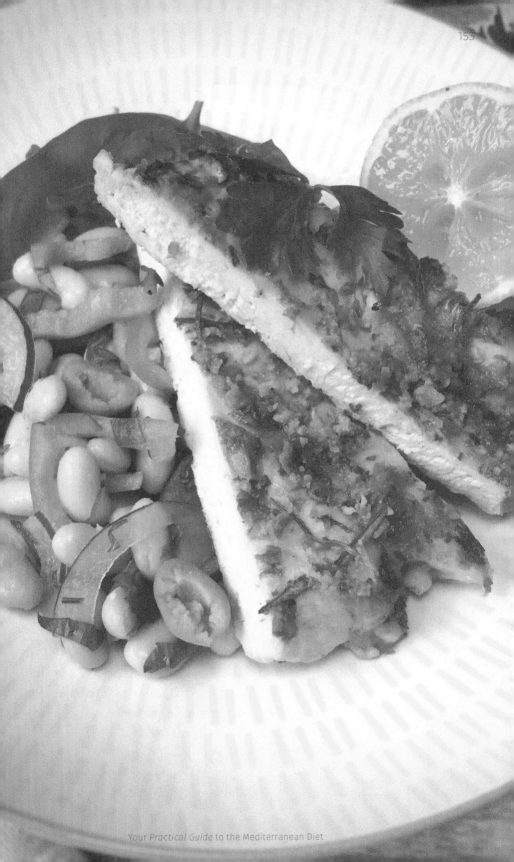

Spanish Smoked Chicken with Almonds

SUITABLE
High Protein

PREP TIME
20 mins

COOK TIME
30 mins

SERVES
2

Nutrition (per serving)	Kcal	Fat	Sat Fat	Carb	Sugar	Fibre	Protein	Salt
	232	6g	0g	16g	1g	6g	31g	2.0g

INGREDIENTS

2 chicken breasts, sliced into strips

7 oz / ½ tin chickpeas

1 tsp olive oil

1 green pepper, thinly sliced

1 red onion, thinly sliced

1 garlic clove, crushed

1 tbsp unblanched almonds, roughly chopped

7 oz / ½ tin chopped tomatoes

1 small bunch parsley, chopped

1 tsp salt

1 tsp sweet smoked paprika (plus 1 pinch)

METHOD

01/ Heat oil in a frying pan until hot. Add chicken breasts & cook over a high heat until golden & seared. Remove from pan. Reduce the heat & add onions & garlic. Stir for 4-5 minutes to soften then add paprika. Stir for 1 minute to release flavor.

02/ Add the pepper strips & return the chicken to the pan. Add the tomatoes then salt & simmer for 8-10 minutes, until the chicken is cooked.

03/ Add chickpeas (reserve a few for serving) & stir to heat them through. Meanwhile, put almonds & reserved chickpeas in a bowl with a pinch of paprika & stir to coat. Stir in parsley and serve the chicken and peppers. Scatter almonds & chickpeas.

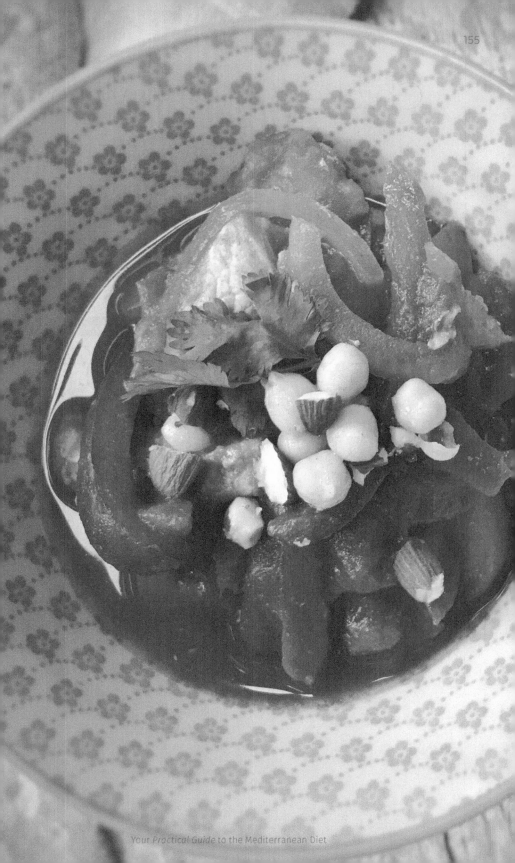

Chicken & Ham with New Potatoes

SUITABLE
Quick

PREP TIME
5 mins

COOK TIME
15 mins

SERVES
2

Nutrition (per serving)	Kcal	Fat	Sat Fat	Carb	Sugar	Fibre	Protein	Salt
	332	12g	3g	30g	2g	4g	28g	3.6g

INGREDIENTS

1 ½ cups / 225g new potatoes, halved if large

⅔ cups / 100g green beans, trimmed and sliced

2 skinless chicken breasts

1 tbsp olive oil

2 slices Parma ham

1 garlic clove, crushed

juice ½ lemon

METHOD

01 / Cook potatoes in boiling salted water for 10-15 minutes, until tender. Add green beans for last 2 minutes. Season chicken breasts.

02 / Heat the oil in a frying pan & add ham. Cook for 2 mins, until crisp. Drain on kitchen paper. Add oil to the pan & cook chicken breasts for 3 minutes each side. Transfer to a plate.

03 / Remove pan from heat & add the garlic & lemon juice. Add the drained beans & potatoes & crumble in ham. Divide between plates & serve.

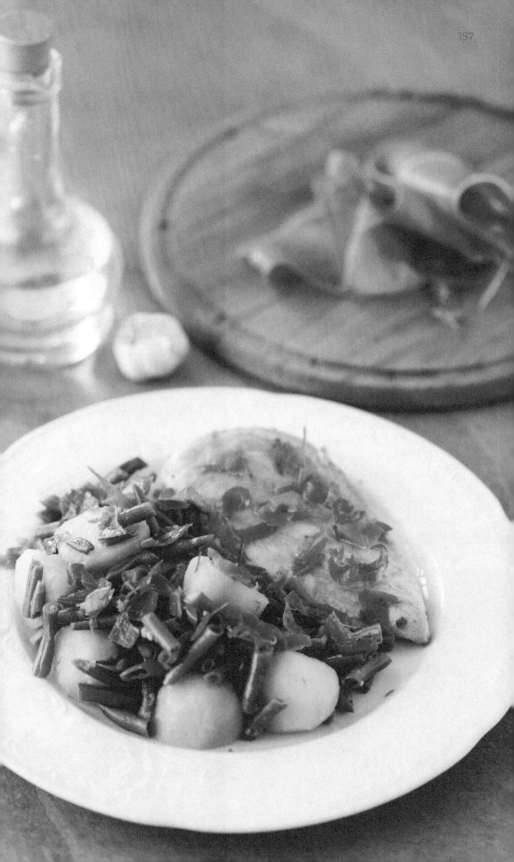

Moroccan Chicken & Sweet Potato Mash

SUITABLE
Quick

PREP TIME
20 mins

COOK TIME
10 mins

SERVES
2

Nutrition (per serving)	Kcal	Fat	Sat Fat	Carb	Sugar	Fibre	Protein	Salt
	384	9g	2g	34g	13g	7g	34g	1.1g

INGREDIENTS

1 ¾ cups / 250g sweet potatoes, cubed

½ tsp ground cinnamon

½ tsp ground cumin

2 chicken breasts

1 tbsp olive oil

½ onion, thinly sliced

1 garlic clove, crushed

⅔ cup / 100ml chicken or vegetable stock

1 tsp clear honey

juice ½ lemon

handful olives, pitted or whole

½ cup / 10g cilantro, leaves chopped

METHOD

01/ Boil the potatoes in salted water for 15 minutes or until tender. Mix the cumin & cinnamon with ground pepper, then sprinkle over the chicken. Heat 1 tbsp oil in a frying pan, then cook the chicken for 3 minutes on each side until golden.

02/ Remove chicken from the pan. Add the onion & garlic & cook for 5 minutes until soft. Add stock, honey, lemon juice & olives, return the chicken to the pan, then simmer for 10 minutes until the chicken is cooked.

03/ Mash the potatoes with 1 tbsp oil & season. Slice each chicken breast & stir the cilantro through the sauce before serving.

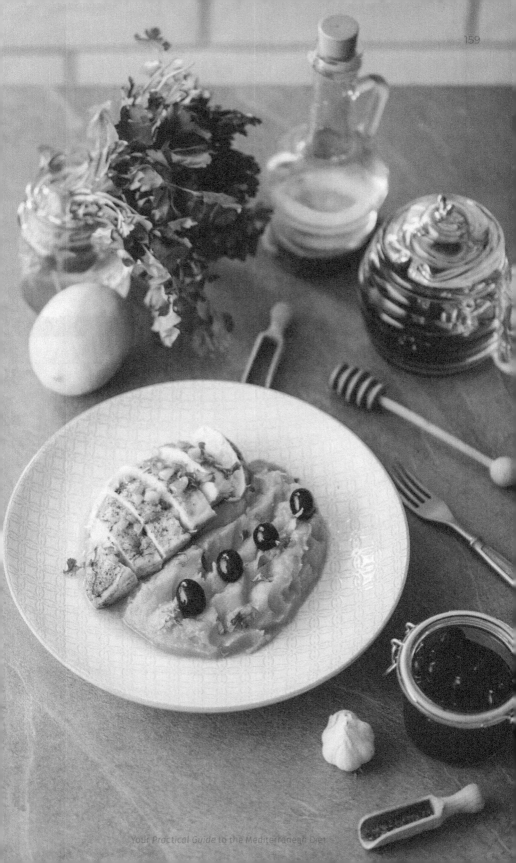

Chicken & Mushroom Cream Bucatini

SUITABLE	**PREP TIME**	**COOK TIME**	**SERVES**
Quick	5 mins	20 mins	2

Nutrition (per serving)	Kcal	Fat	Sat Fat	Carb	Sugar	Fibre	Protein	Salt
	465	13g	4g	53g	9g	3g	40g	1.5g

INGREDIENTS

1 tbsp butter

1 tbsp flour

1 ⅕ cup / 300ml milk

1 tsp salt

2 chicken breast, sliced

1 tsp olive oil

2 cups / 150g chestnut mushrooms, sliced

1 cup / 200g dried bucatini (or use wholemeal spaghetti)

basil, to serve (optional)

METHOD

01 / Cook pasta as per packet instructions.

02 / In a small saucepan, add the flour, butter & milk. Stir for 6-7 minutes until melted, mixed & thickened.

03 / In a frying pan, add the chicken slices. Heat for 3-4 minutes and then add the mushrooms. Heat for another 3-4 minutes until the chicken is cooked through. Drain the spaghetti, add the sauce & stir through the chicken and mushrooms. Serve immediately.

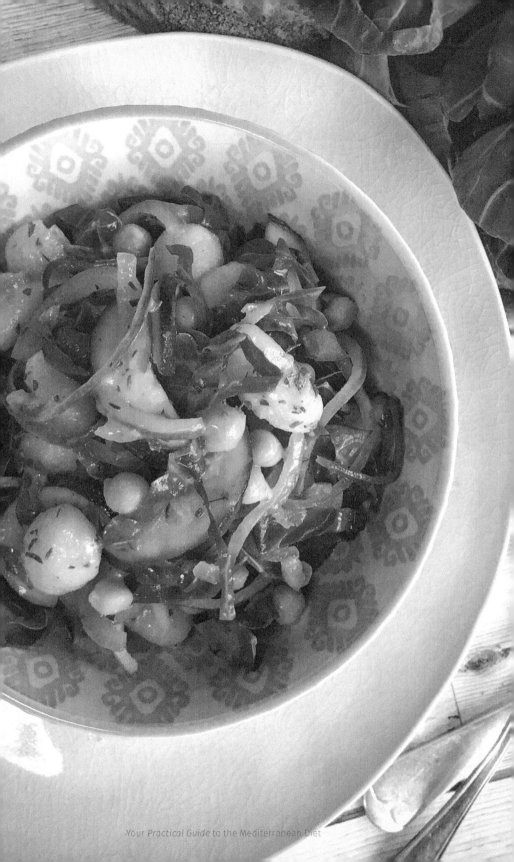

Chicken and Almond Casserole

SUITABLE

Quick

PREP TIME

5 mins

COOK TIME

20 mins

SERVES

2

Nutrition (per serving)	Kcal	Fat	Sat Fat	Carb	Sugar	Fibre	Protein	Salt
	455	19g	2g	32g	11g	10g	37g	2.3g

INGREDIENTS

1 tsp olive oil

2 chicken breasts, sliced

1 onion, halved and sliced

1 green pepper, sliced

3 tbsp chickpeas

14 oz / 1 tin chopped tomatoes

1 ¼ cup / 300ml vegetable stock

1 tsp salt

1 tsp honey

1 tsp fennel seeds

1 tbsp whole almonds, roughly chopped

fresh parsley to serve *(optional)*

METHOD

01/ In a saucepan, heat the oil. Add the onion and stir for 3-4 minutes, until soft. Add the chicken breast slices and turn the heat up to color them. Add the pepper, chickpeas and tin tomatoes. Bring to a simmer, add the honey, fennel and salt and stir. Cover with a lid and simmer gently for 20 minutes, until the chicken is cooked.

02/ Serve immediately between two bowls with parsley. Sprinkle over the chopped almonds.

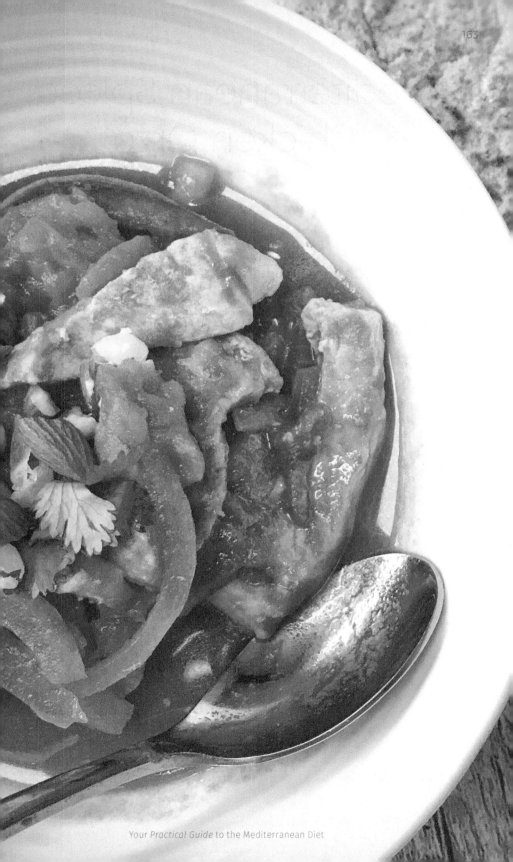

Mediterranean Spiced Chicken Orzo

SUITABLE

High Protein

PREP TIME

5 mins

COOK TIME

45 mins

SERVES

2

Nutrition (per serving)	Kcal	Fat	Sat Fat	Carb	Sugar	Fibre	Protein	Salt
	505	10g	2g	53g	6g	4g	53g	1.6g

INGREDIENTS

4 skinless chicken thighs

¾ cup / 150g orzo

1 tsp olive oil

½ onion, chopped finely

1 red pepper, sliced

1 green pepper, sliced

14 oz / 1 tin of chopped tomatoes

1 tsp salt

METHOD

01 / Pre-heat the oven to 400F (200C) and grease a medium casserole dish.

02 / In a saucepan, heat the oil. Add the chicken thighs & brown for 2-3 minutes on both sides. Add to the casserole dish.

03 / Lower the heat and add the onion & peppers. Stir until softened. Add the salt & tomatoes and bring to a boil. Pour over the chicken & bake for 30 minutes until cooked.

04 / Towards the end of the cooking time, cook the orzo as per packet instructions. Drain and mix with the chicken just before serving.

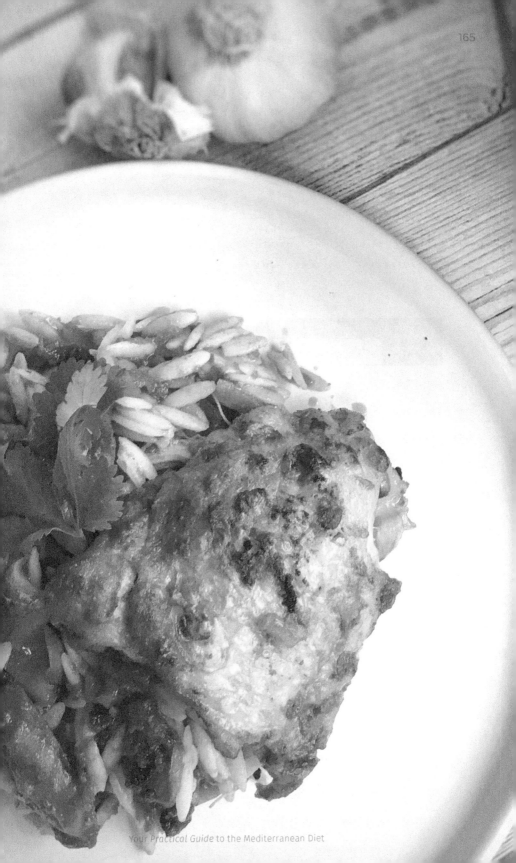

Lemon & Garlic Chicken

SUITABLE

High Protein

PREP TIME

5 mins

COOK TIME

40 mins

SERVES

2

Nutrition (per serving)	Kcal	Fat	Sat Fat	Carb	Sugar	Fibre	Protein	Salt
	278	11g	2g	8g	2g	2g	42g	3.1g

INGREDIENTS

1 tsp olive oil

4 skinless chicken thighs

1 onion, halved and sliced

2 garlic cloves, crushed

1 lemon, zest only

1 preserved lemon, sliced

1 celery stalk, sliced

5-6 chestnut mushrooms, sliced

handful of black olives

METHOD

01/ Pre-heat the oven to 400F (200C) and grease a medium casserole dish.

02/ Massage the lemon zest, oil and crushed garlic into the chicken thighs. Place the sliced onion and celery on the bottom of the casserole dish with the preserved lemon. Place the chicken thighs on top and bake in the oven for 30 minutes.

03/ Remove from the oven and add the mushrooms and olives to the chicken. Continue to cook for a further 10 minutes, until the chicken is cooked and the mushrooms softened.

04/ Serve with either rice or potato side dish.

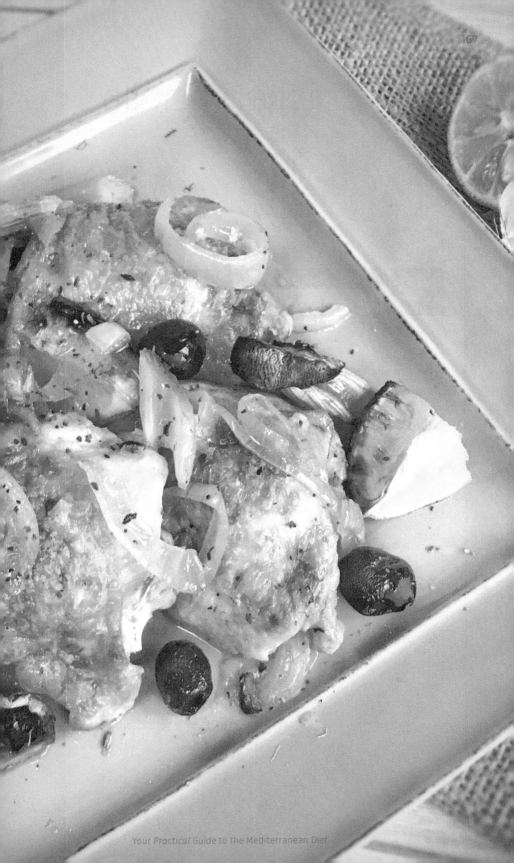

Chicken Paella

SUITABLE

High Protein

PREP TIME

10 mins

COOK TIME

40 mins

SERVES

4

Nutrition (per serving)	Kcal	Fat	Sat Fat	Carb	Sugar	Fibre	Protein	Salt
	563	16g	5g	62g	5g	7g	38g	1.9g

INGREDIENTS

1 tbsp olive oil

2 chicken breast fillets, cut into chunks

2 onions, finely sliced

1 garlic clove, crushed

1 cup / 140g cooking chorizo, sliced

1 tsp turmeric

pinch of saffron

1 tsp paprika

1 ½ cups / 300g paella rice

3 ½ cups / 850ml hot vegetable stock

1 cup / 200g frozen peas

½ small pack parsley, chopped, to serve

METHOD

01/ Heat the oil in a frying pan over a high heat. Add the chicken and brown all over and transfer to a plate. Reduce the heat to low, add the onions and cook slowly until softened, about 10 minutes.

02/ Add the garlic, stir for 1 minute, then add chorizo and fry until it releases its oils. Add spices and rice and stir for about 2 minutes, then pour in the hot stock. Bring to a boil, add the chicken and simmer for 20 minutes, stirring occasionally.

03/ Add the peas and simmer for 5 minutes until the rice is cooked and the chicken is tender. Season well and serve with chopped parsley.

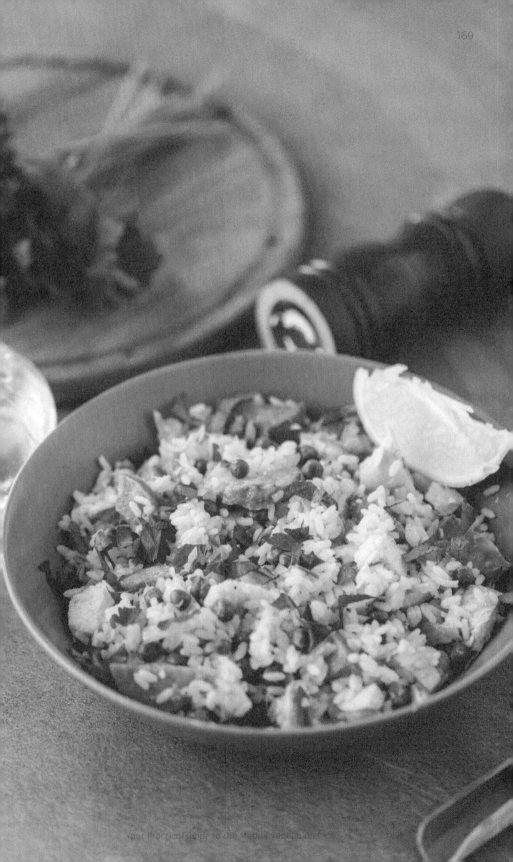

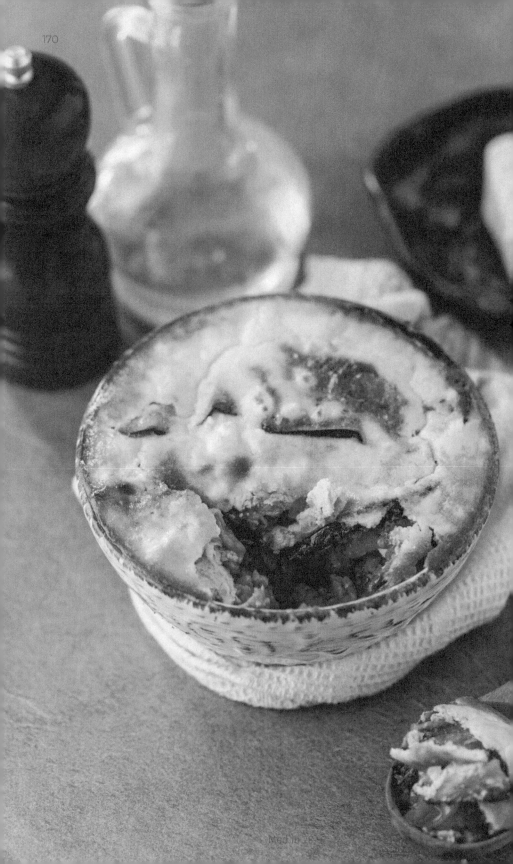

Meat

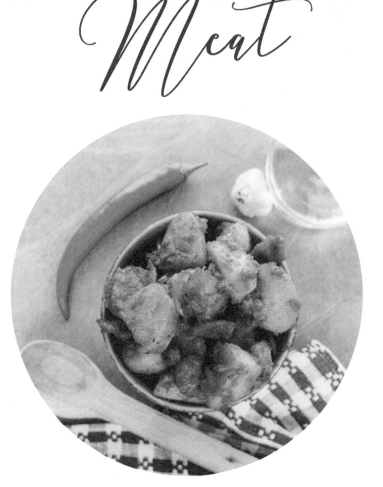

Spanish Chorizo & Chickpea Soup

SUITABLE

Quick

PREP TIME

5 mins

COOK TIME

10 mins

SERVES

2

Nutrition (per serving)	Kcal	Fat	Sat Fat	Carb	Sugar	Fibre	Protein	Salt
	548	25g	8g	48g	2g	9g	28g	2.7g

INGREDIENTS

14 oz / 400g can chopped tomatoes

⅔ cup / 110g pack of chorizo sausage

1 ½ cups / 140g wedge Savoy cabbage

sprinkling dried chilli flakes

14 oz / 410g can chickpeas, drained and rinsed

1 vegetable stock cube

brown bread, to serve

METHOD

01/ Put a medium pan on the heat and tip in the tomatoes, followed by a can of water. While the tomatoes are heating, quickly chop the chorizo into chunky pieces (removing any skin) and shred the cabbage.

02/ Pile the chorizo and cabbage into the pan with the chilli flakes and chickpeas, then crumble in the stock cube. Stir well, cover and leave to bubble over a high heat for 6 mins or until the cabbage is just tender. Ladle into bowls and serve with bread.

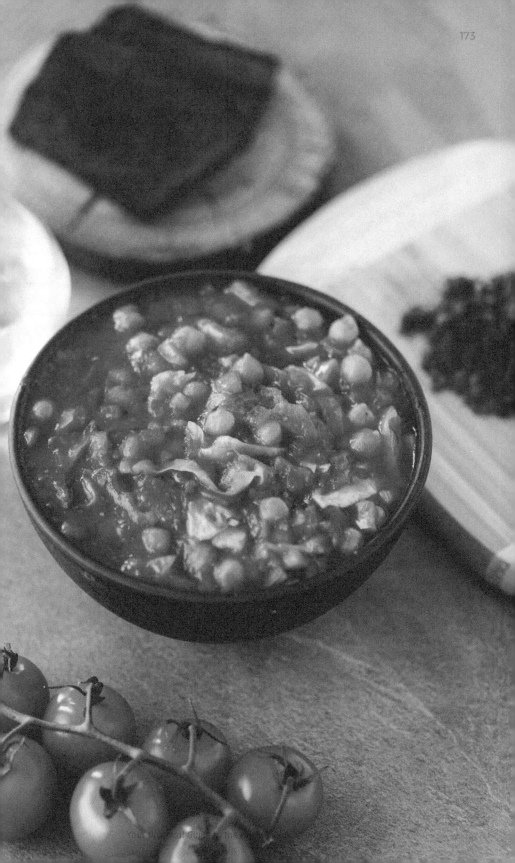

Moussaka

SUITABLE

Quick

PREP TIME

10 mins

COOK TIME

20 mins

SERVES

2

Nutrition (per serving)	Kcal	Fat	Sat Fat	Carb	Sugar	Fibre	Protein	Salt
	370	11g	2g	30g	7g	6g	38g	0.3g

INGREDIENTS

- ½ lb / 250g lean minced beef
- ½ eggplant / aubergine
- ⅓ cup / 75g Greek yogurt
- 1 egg, beaten
- 1 tbsp / 15g feta cheese
- 7 oz / 200g can chopped tomatoes with garlic and herbs
- 2 tbsp sun-dried tomato purée
- 1 cup / 175g boiled potatoes

METHOD

01 / Heat the grill to high and brown the beef in a pan for 5 minutes. Meanwhile, prick the eggplant with a fork and microwave on high for 3-5 minutes until soft. Mix the yogurt, egg & feta together, then add seasoning.

02 / Stir the tomatoes, purée & potatoes in with the beef, season and heat through. Slice the cooked eggplant and arrange on top of the beef mixture. Pour the yogurt mixture over the eggplant, smooth and grill until the topping is golden.

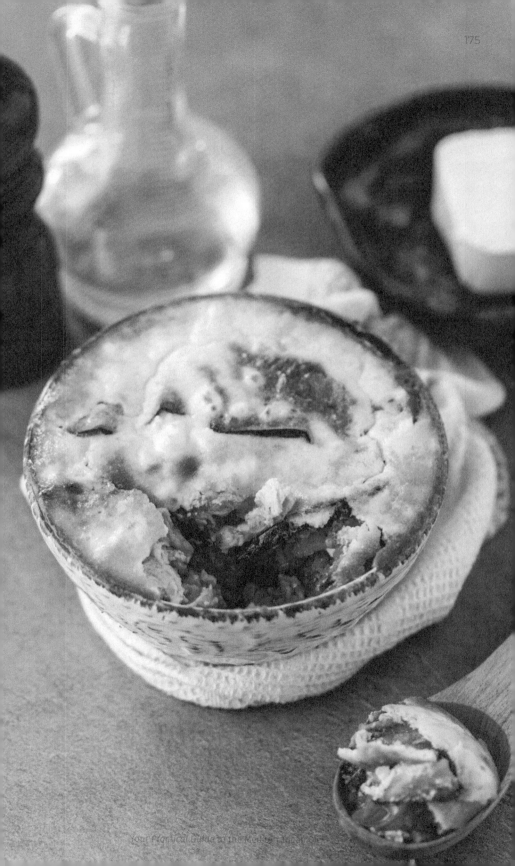

Spanish Chorizo Hot Pot

SUITABLE

Quick

PREP TIME

5 mins

COOK TIME

15 mins

SERVES

2

Nutrition (per serving)	Kcal	Fat	Sat Fat	Carb	Sugar	Fibre	Protein	Salt
	285	9g	3g	9g	4g	5g	9g	0.7g

INGREDIENTS

1 tsp olive oil

1 onion, chopped finely

2 green bell peppers, sliced

½ cup / 70-90g of chopped chorizo

14 oz / 1 tin of chopped tomatoes

1 tsp dried oregano

9-10 new potatoes, cubed and steamed

cilantro, chopped, to serve

METHOD

01/ In a saucepan, heat the oil. Add onion & stir for 3-4 minutes, until soft. Add chopped chorizo & cook for 4-5 minutes. Add the pepper and cook for another 4-5 minutes until softened a little.

02/ Add tomatoes, potatoes & oregano to the pan & simmer. Cook for 5 minutes until everything is hot and cooked through. Serve with cilantro.

Notes:

Add a slice of wholemeal bread or protein (chicken, pork, fish) to make it a more substantial meal. If adding meat, use slightly less chorizo.

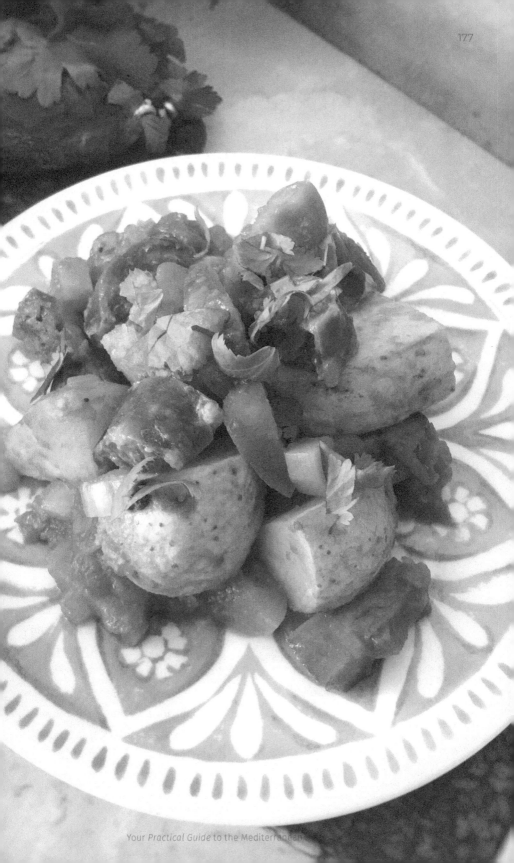

Lamb and Pine Nut Rice Bowl

SUITABLE
High Protein

PREP TIME
5 mins

COOK TIME
30 mins

SERVES
2

Nutrition (per serving)	Kcal	Fat	Sat Fat	Carb	Sugar	Fibre	Protein	Salt
	557	21g	5g	54g	9g	6g	37g	0.2g

INGREDIENTS

- 1 ½ cups / 250g ready cooked basmati rice pouch
- 1 tsp olive oil
- 1 onion, chopped finely
- 1 garlic clove, crushed
- 1 small zucchini / courgette, sliced or cubed
- 1 medium carrot, sliced or cubed
- 14 oz / 1 tin of chopped tomatoes
- 1 tsp salt
- 7 oz / 200g lamb leg/neck fillet, cut into cubes
- 1 tbsp pine nuts

METHOD

01/ In a saucepan, heat the oil. When hot, flash fry the lamb pieces until browned all over. Remove from the pan and keep warm.

02/ Lower the heat, and add the onion and garlic. Cook for 4-5 minutes until softened. Add the carrots and cook for a further 5-6 minutes until slightly soft. Add the zucchini and when coated in oil, add the tomatoes and salt. Stir everything together until softened and simmer.

03/ Return the lamb back to the pan and cook for a further 5-6 minutes. Serve the lamb with rice, cooked with turmeric.

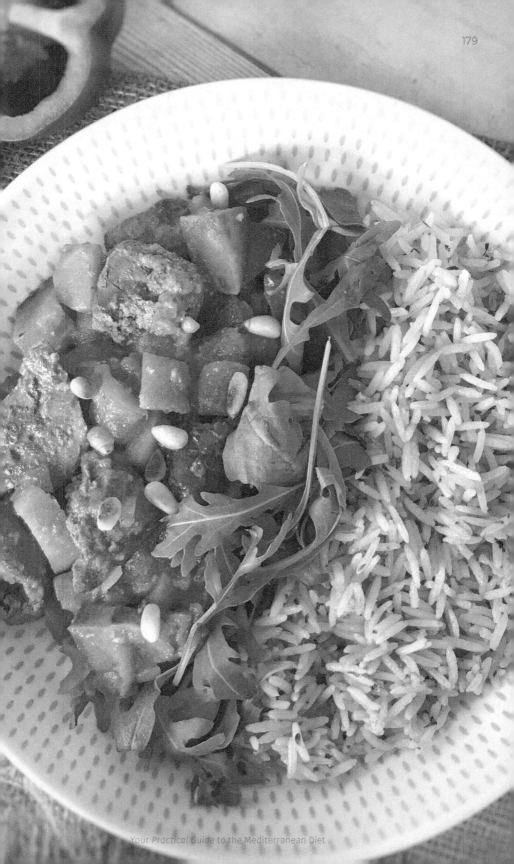

Lamb & Beetroot Stew

SUITABLE
High Protein

PREP TIME
10 mins

COOK TIME
30 mins

SERVES
2

Nutrition (per serving)	Kcal	Fat	Sat Fat	Carb	Sugar	Fibre	Protein	Salt
	510	17g	7g	65g	13g	11g	27g	3.1g

INGREDIENTS

7 oz / 200g lamb neck fillet

3 tbsp olive oil

1 red onion, halved and sliced

1 garlic clove, crushed

2 medium carrots, halved & sliced

1 medium beetroot, peeled & cut

1 tsp cumin

½ tsp ground cilantro

½ tsp cinnamon

½ tsp turmeric

2 handfuls of cabbage, shredded

1 ⅔ cups / 400ml vegetable stock

1 tbsp pumpkin seeds

¾ cups / 150g couscous

1 ¼ cups / 300ml vegetable stock

1 tsp chopped rosemary

½ tsp dried tarragon

METHOD

01/ Heat 1 tbsp of oil in a saucepan & add onion & garlic. Stir over medium heat for 4-5 minutes until softened. Add beetroot, carrot & spices. Cook on a low heat, adding the stock & placing the lid on half way.

02/ When vegetables are almost cooked, heat 1 tbsp of oil in a frying pan. When hot, add lamb pieces & fry on high heat until colored on all sides. Boil vegetable stock for the couscous. Stir the herbs into the couscous & pour over stock. Cover with cling film & leave to absorb.

03/ Add lamb to the vegetables & shredded greens & stir until the vegetables are cooked. Fluff up couscous with a fork and serve on 2 plates. Spoon lamb & vegetables on top & sprinkle with pumpkin seeds.

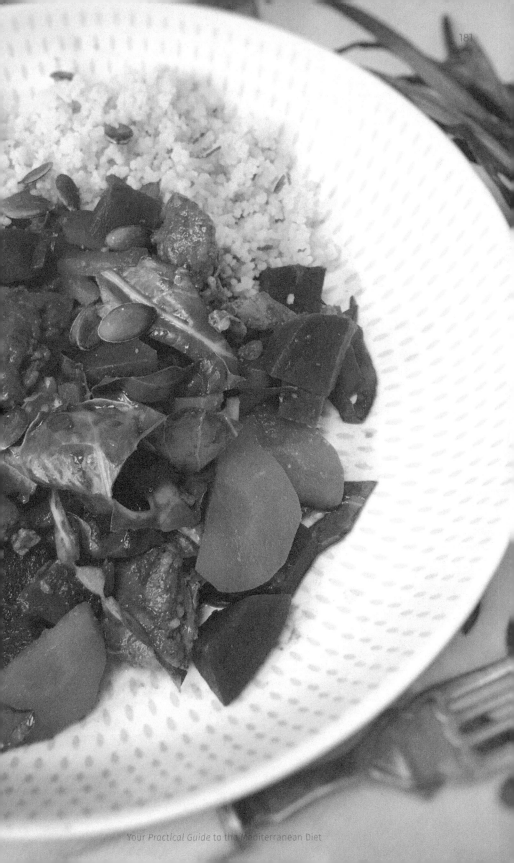

Avocado, Basil & Smoked Ham

SUITABLE
Quick

PREP TIME
5 mins

COOK TIME
15 mins

SERVES
2

Nutrition (per serving)	Kcal	Fat	Sat Fat	Carb	Sugar	Fibre	Protein	Salt
	421	16g	3g	45g	2g	12g	26g	2.3g

INGREDIENTS

1 avocado

5-6 fresh basil leaves

½ lemon, juice only

1 garlic clove

¼ tsp salt

1 cup / 200g wholewheat pasta

1 tbsp pumpkin seeds

handful of smoked ham chunks

2 handfuls of rocket leaves / arugula

METHOD

01/ Heat a large pan of water and cook the pasta, as instructed on the packet.

02/ In a blender, add the basil leaves, avocado and lemon juice and blend until you have created a smooth sauce.

03/ Drain the pasta and stir in the avocado sauce. Stir through the ham chunks and leave to cool a little.

04/ Add arugula and divide between 2 bowls. Sprinkle with pumpkin seeds and serve.

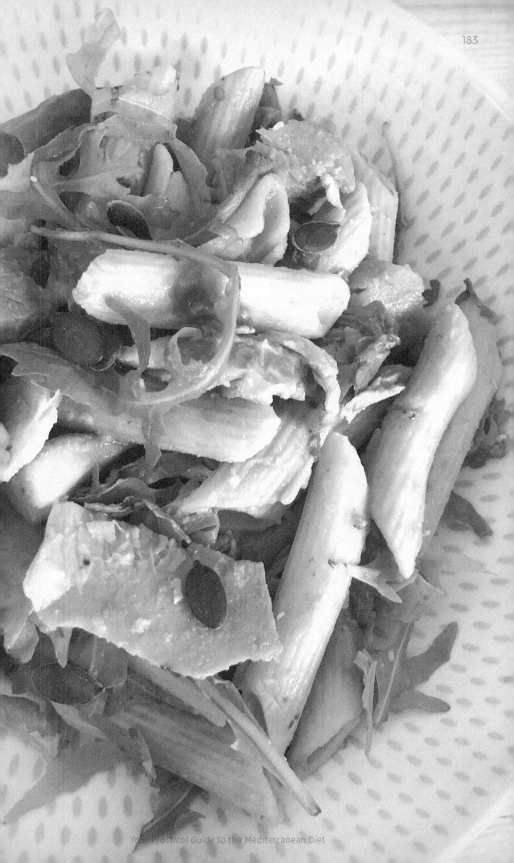

Pork, Zucchini Fritters & Apple Sauce

SUITABLE
Quick

PREP TIME
5 mins

COOK TIME
20 mins

SERVES
2

Nutrition (per serving)	Kcal	Fat	Sat Fat	Carb	Sugar	Fibre	Protein	Salt
	365	16g	5g	21g	9g	3g	33g	0.7g

INGREDIENTS

1 tsp olive oil

2 spring onions, sliced

1 medium zucchini / courgette, grated

1 egg

2 tbsp self-raising flour

1 tbsp milk

2 tbsp grated parmesan

1 tsp olive oil

2 pork loin chops *(fat removed)*

1 apple, sliced

2 tbsp apple sauce

sunflower seeds & rocket / arugula, to serve

METHOD

01/ In a frying pan, heat the oil. Mix the zucchini, flour, egg, cheese & onion. Place dollops of the mixture in the oil. Cook over a medium heat on both sides, until golden. Remove from pan & keep warm.

02/ Heat the oil in the pan for the pork, or alternatively, cook the pork chops under a grill whilst you are cooking the fritters to save time. Cook the pork chops for 5-6 minutes on both sides depending on the thickness of your meat.

03/ To serve, divide the fritters between 2 plates, add the pork chops, some fresh apple slices and some apple sauce. Serve with green salad or steamed vegetables.

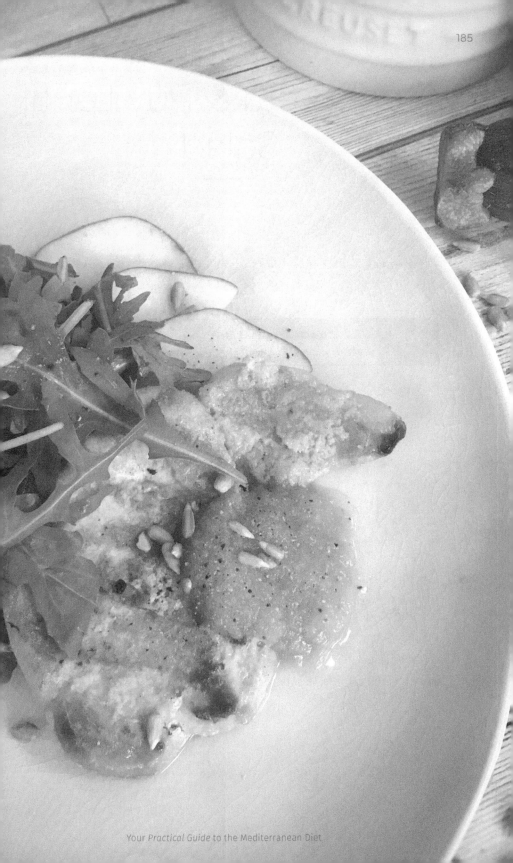

Steak, Feta & Puy Lentil Salad

SUITABLE

High Protein

PREP TIME

15 mins

COOK TIME

25 mins

SERVES

2

Nutrition (per serving)	Kcal	Fat	Sat Fat	Carb	Sugar	Fibre	Protein	Salt
	397	19g	8g	30g	6g	7g	27g	1.8g

INGREDIENTS

½ tbsp olive oil

1 red onion, halved and sliced

1 rump or sirloin steak

⅓ cup / 50g feta cheese, cut into small cubes

1 red bell pepper, cut into small dices

handful of baby spinach leaves

1 ¼ cup / 250g pouch of ready cooked puy lentils

1 tbsp balsamic dressing

salt and pepper, for seasoning

small handful of cress, to serve.

METHOD

01 / Heat a griddle pan until very hot. Rub the steak with the oil, salt & pepper. Sear the steak on both sides in the griddle pan. Add the onion to the pan with the steak & cook for roughly 4-5 minutes on each side (depending on how thick your steak is & how you like it cooked) & until the onion is soft. Leave steak to rest & remove the onions.

02 / Mix the rest of the ingredients together in a bowl. Slice the steak thinly and stir through the salad with the onions.

03 / Divide between 2 plates, drizzle with the balsamic dressing and top with the cress.

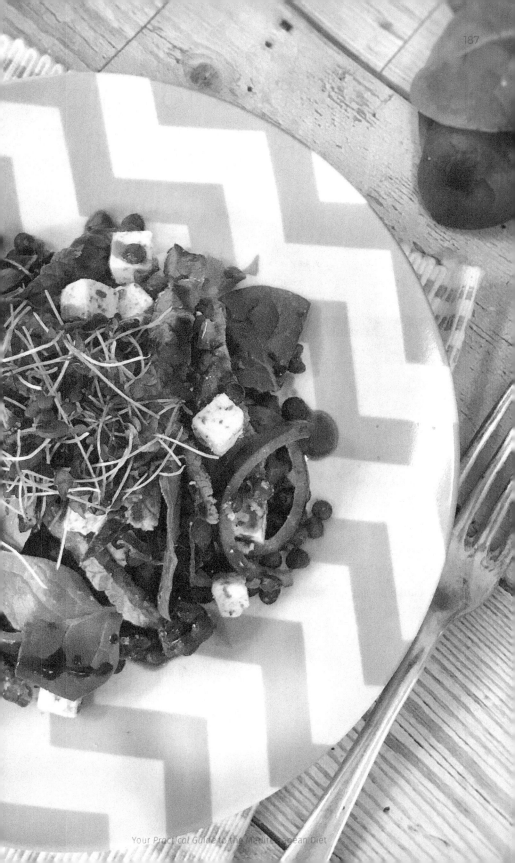

Meatball & Tomato Risotto

SUITABLE
Quick

PREP TIME
5 mins

COOK TIME
25 mins

SERVES
2

Nutrition (per serving)	Kcal	Fat	Sat Fat	Carb	Sugar	Fibre	Protein	Salt
	549	13g	5g	46g	5g	2g	18g	2.2g

INGREDIENTS

1 tsp olive oil

½ onion, chopped finely

7-8 beef meatballs

1 cup / 200g arborio rice

14 oz / 1 tin of chopped tomatoes

1 tsp salt

1 tsp dried oregano

1 ⅔ cups / 400ml vegetable stock

fresh basil to serve

METHOD

01 / Pre-heat the oven to 400 F (200C) and grease a baking tin. Add the meatballs to the tin and bake in the oven for 15 minutes, until cooked.

02 / Meanwhile, in a saucepan, heat the oil. Add the onion and stir for 3-4 minutes, until soft. Add the arborio rice and stir to coat with the oil. Add the tin tomatoes, salt, oregano and stock. Stir well and bring to a simmer.

03 / Place a lid on the saucepan and simmer over a low heat for 20 minutes until the rice is cooked.

04 / Stir through the meatballs and divide between 2 plates. Serve with torn basil leaves.

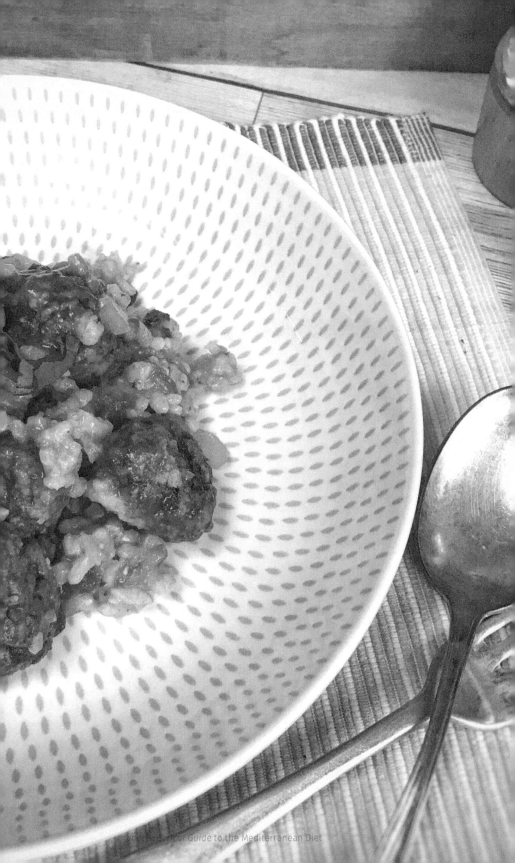

Lamb & Feta Orzo Bake

SUITABLE
Quick

PREP TIME
5 mins

COOK TIME
20 mins

SERVES
2

Nutrition (per serving)	Kcal	Fat	Sat Fat	Carb	Sugar	Fibre	Protein	Salt
	468	23g	8g	48g	5g	3g	23g	1.5g

INGREDIENTS

8 lamb meatballs

¾ cup / 150g dried orzo

1 ½ cups / 150g chestnut mushrooms, sliced

⅔ cups / 100g feta cheese, cubed

juice of 1 Lemon

bunch of mint leaves, shredded

2 handfuls of baby spinach leaves

1 tsp olive oil

METHOD

01/ In a saucepan, heat the oil. Add the meatballs and brown all over.

02/ Add the mushrooms and cook over a medium heat. Cook until softened and the meatballs cooked thoroughly.

03/ Meanwhile, cook the orzo in a saucepan of water, as per packet instructions.

04/ When ready to serve, tip the pasta into the saucepan with the lemon juice, feta and mint.

05/ Divide between 2 plates and add the baby spinach.

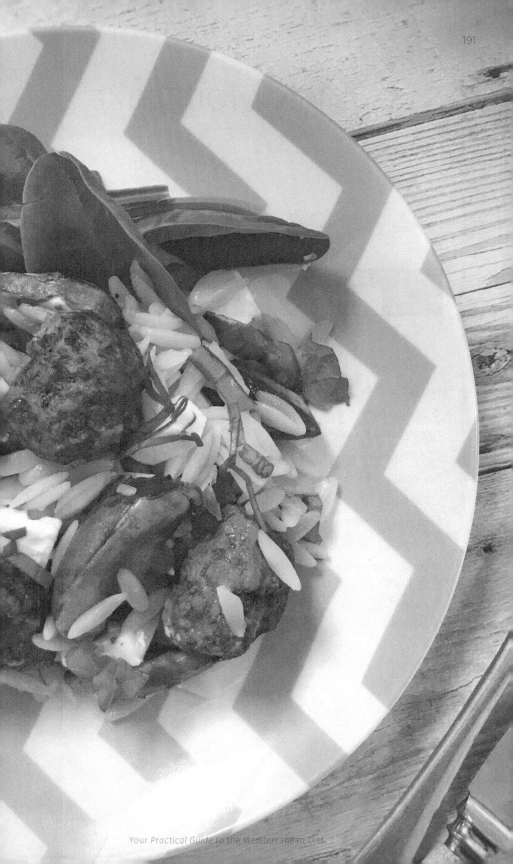

Quick Moussaka

SUITABLE

Quick

PREP TIME

10 mins

COOK TIME

20 mins

SERVES

2

Nutrition (per serving)	Kcal	Fat	Sat Fat	Carb	Sugar	Fibre	Protein	Salt
	577	27g	12g	46g	6g	8g	41g	2.8g

INGREDIENTS

1 tbsp olive oil

½ onion, finely chopped

1 garlic clove, finely chopped

9 oz / 250g lean beef mince

7 oz / 200g can chopped tomatoes

1 tbsp tomato purée

1 tsp ground cinnamon

7 oz / 200g can chickpeas

⅔ cup / 100g pack feta cheese, crumbled

dried mint

brown bread, to serve

METHOD

01 / Heat the oil in a pan. Add the onion and garlic and fry until soft. Add the mince and fry for 3-4 minutes until browned.

02 / Tip the tomatoes into the pan and stir in the tomato purée and cinnamon, then season. Leave the mince to simmer for 20 minutes. Add the chickpeas halfway through.

03 / Sprinkle the feta and dried mint over the mince. Serve with toasted bread.

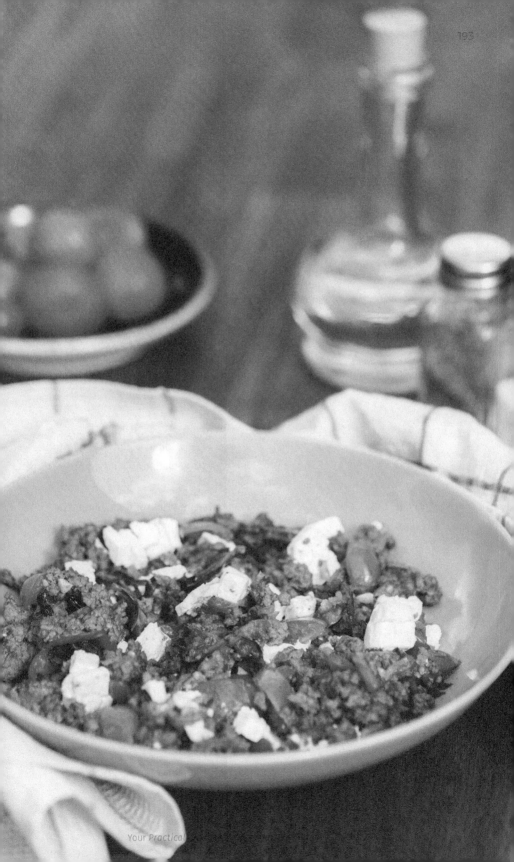

Patatas Bravas with Chorizo

SUITABLE

/

PREP TIME

10 mins

COOK TIME

40 mins

SERVES

2

Nutrition (per serving)	Kcal	Fat	Sat Fat	Carb	Sugar	Fibre	Protein	Salt
	551	31g	10g	48g	7g	8g	21g	2.3g

INGREDIENTS

1 tbsp olive oil

½ onion, chopped

1 garlic clove, sliced

1 red chilli, chopped

pinch cayanne chilli pepper

pinch smoked paprika

7 oz / 200g can chopped tomatoes

3 ½ cups / 500g new potatoes, halved or quartered

4-5 oz / 125g small cooking chorizo

METHOD

01/ Heat oil in a pan, fry the onion, garlic & chilli until the onion softens, then stir in the pepper & paprika. Add the tomatoes & simmer the mixture for 20 minutes until it's a thick paste. Season well.

02/ Meanwhile, steam the potatoes for 10 mins and cook the chorizo in a frying pan to slowly release some of its oil. Tip off the excess red oil and add 1 tbsp olive oil. Add potatoes and fry everything together. Tip into a bowl, season the sauce and spoon it over the potatoes & chorizo to serve.

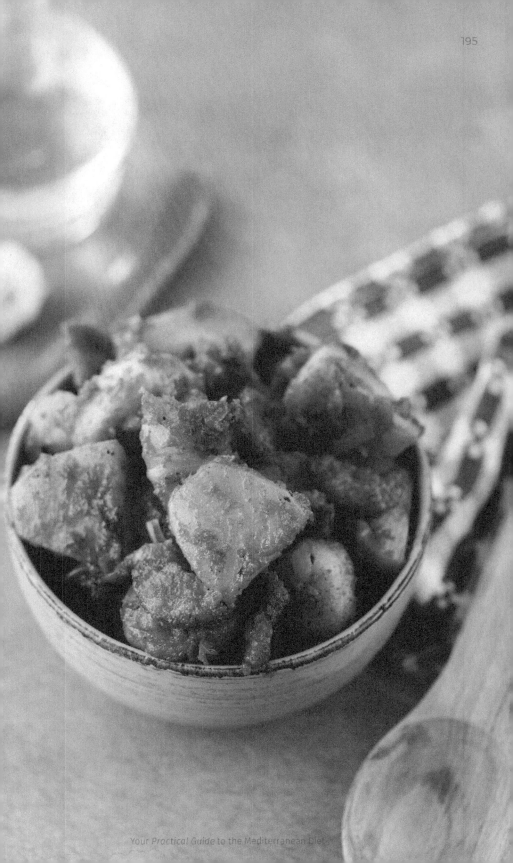

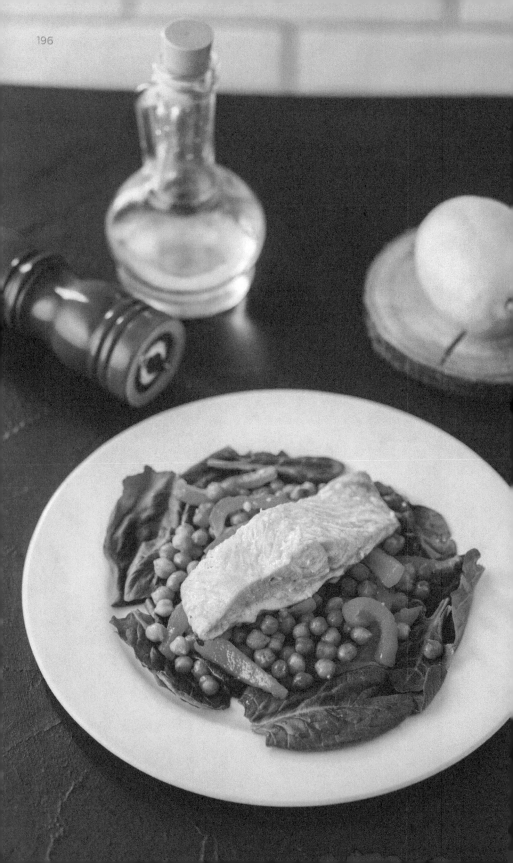

Fish

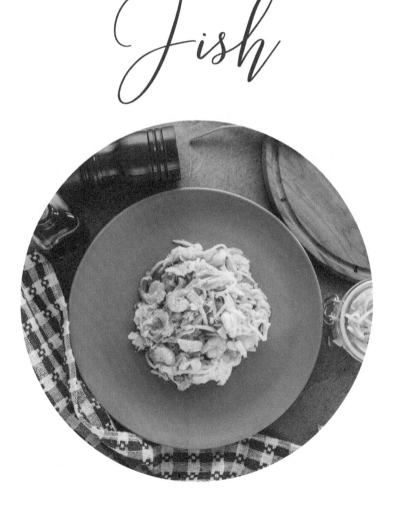

Haddock Risotto

SUITABLE
High Protein

PREP TIME
10 mins

COOK TIME
40 mins

SERVES
2

Nutrition (per serving)	Kcal	Fat	Sat Fat	Carb	Sugar	Fibre	Protein	Salt
	613	16g	2g	56g	6g	3g	45g	3.1g

INGREDIENTS

1 tbsp olive oil

1 large leek, thinly sliced

¾ cup / 150g risotto rice, such as arborio or carnaroli

1 ½ cups / 350ml vegetable stock

½ cup / 125ml milk

9-10 oz / 280g smoked haddock, skinned and cut into large chunks

2 tbsp crème fraîche

1 ⅔ cups / 50g baby spinach

METHOD

01/ Heat oven to 400F (200C). Heat the oil in an oven-proof dish over a medium heat. Cook the leek for 4-5 minutes, until just tender. Add the rice and stir for 2 extra minutes.

02/ Add the stock and milk, bring to a boil and simmer for 5 minutes. Add the haddock on top. Cover with foil and bake in the oven for 18 minutes until the rice is tender.

03/ Add the crème fraîche and spinach and season. Cover the pan again and leave to rest out of the oven for 3 minutes before serving.

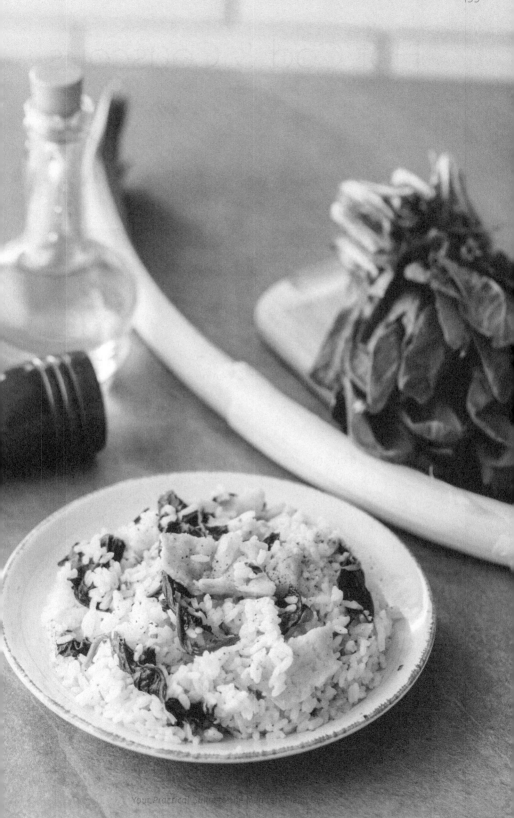

Hot Cod & Couscous

SUITABLE

Quick

PREP TIME

5 mins

COOK TIME

20 mins

SERVES

2

Nutrition (per serving)	Kcal	Fat	Sat Fat	Carb	Sugar	Fibre	Protein	Salt
	504	9g	1g	65g	5g	5g	38g	0.8g

INGREDIENTS

1 tbsp olive oil

½ red onion, sliced

1 garlic clove, chopped

2 tsp harissa paste

2 cod fillets

⅛ cup / 20g dried breadcrumbs

½ lemon, zest & juice

⅔ cup / 125g couscous

⅚ cup / 200ml hot vegetable stock

bunch of parsley, chopped

METHOD

01 / Heat oil in a frying pan. Add onion and cook for 5 minutes until softened. Add garlic and cook for 2-3 minutes more. Season and set aside.

02 / Meanwhile, heat the grill to medium. Spread harissa paste on top of the fish, then sprinkle over the breadcrumbs and lemon zest. Grill for 10-12 minutes until the fish is just cooked.

03 / While the fish is cooking, put the couscous in a bowl, pour over hot stock and cover with cling film. Leave for 5-10 minutes to absorb, then fluff with a fork.

04 / Add lemon juice and parsley to couscous with onion and garlic. Serve in bowls, topped with the fish.

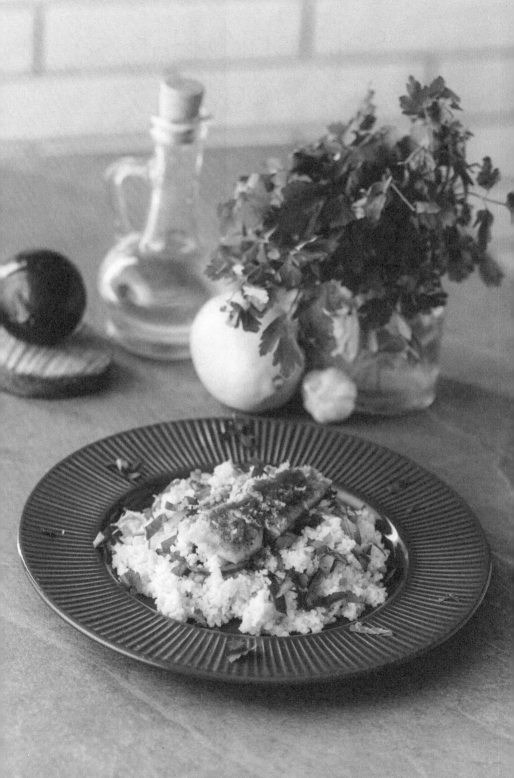

Salmon & Harissa Yogurt

SUITABLE
Quick

PREP TIME
15 mins

COOK TIME
10 mins

SERVES
2

Nutrition (per serving)	Kcal	Fat	Sat Fat	Carb	Sugar	Fibre	Protein	Salt
	540	13g	3g	55g	14g	3g	50g	0.3g

INGREDIENTS

½ cup / 100g couscous

2 tbsp sultanas

small bunch cilantro, chopped

1 tsp ground cinnamon, plus a pinch

⅚ cup / 200ml hot vegetable stock

1 tbsp honey

1 tbsp olive oil

2 salmon fillets

1 tbsp harissa paste

⅔ cup / 170g Greek yogurt

METHOD

01 / Heat the grill. Put the couscous, sultanas, most of the cilantro, 1 tsp cinnamon & seasoning into a bowl. Pour over hot vegetable stock and set aside for 5 minutes.

02 / Mix together cinnamon, honey & oil. Put salmon on a baking tray, spread over the honey mixture and season. Cook under grill for 8 minutes until the fish is cooked through.

03 / Meanwhile, swirl together the harissa and yogurt. Fluff up the couscous with a fork and serve with the fish and yogurt. Sprinkle with the remaining cilantro.

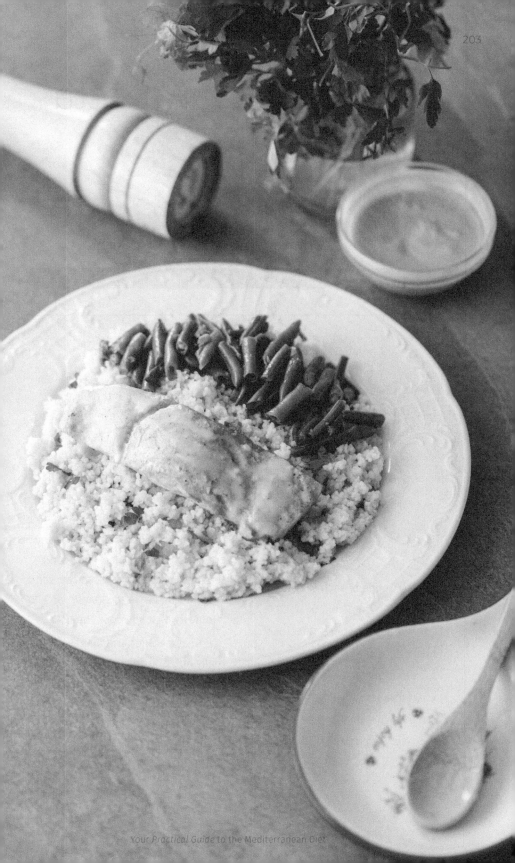

Sea Bass Ciambotta

SUITABLE

Quick

PREP TIME

10 mins

COOK TIME

20 mins

SERVES

2

Nutrition (per serving)	Kcal	Fat	Sat Fat	Carb	Sugar	Fibre	Protein	Salt
	205	3g	1g	18g	5g	7g	29g	1.3g

INGREDIENTS

4 small sea bass fillets

1 tbsp olive oil

½ lemon, zest only

pinch salt

lemon slices to serve

1 tsp olive oil

1 onion, halved and sliced

1 garlic clove, crushed

5-6 baby peppers, each cut into 4

5-6 oz / 150g cannellini beans,

7 oz / ½ tin of chopped tomatoes

½ tsp salt

1 tsp dried oregano & thyme

1 tsp red wine vinegar

1 tsp balsamic vinegar

1 tsp celery seeds

METHOD

01/ Rub the fish with the olive oil, salt & lemon zest. Leave to one side.

02/ Heat the olive oil in a saucepan and add the onion & garlic. Stir for 3-4 minutes until softened. Add the peppers and stir for a further 3-4 minutes. You don't want to cook these until they are too soft as they are better with a little crunch. Add the tin tomatoes, beans, spices, salt and vinegar. Leave to simmer for 9-10 minutes whilst you cook the fish.

03/ Heat a grill or griddle pan until really hot. Starting skin side down, cook the fish over or under a heat for 2-3 minutes each side. Leave the skin side to crisp up as much as you can.

04/ Serve with new potatoes, pasta, polenta or bread.

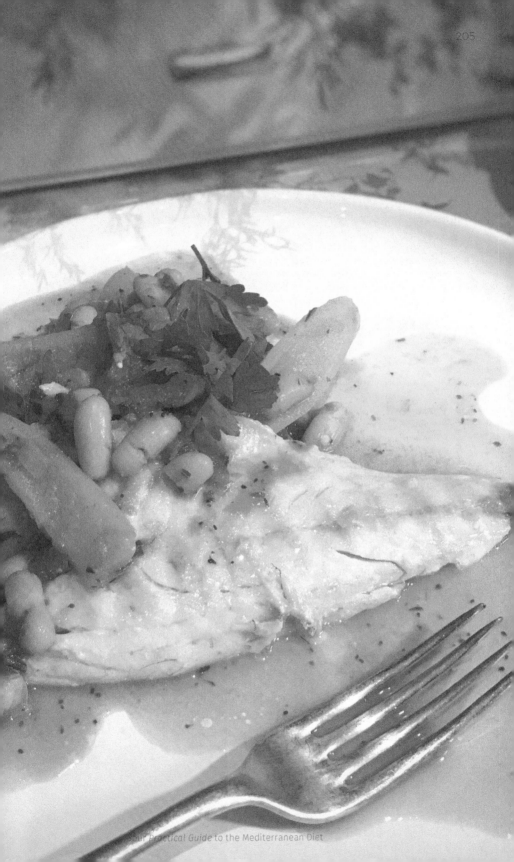

Salmon with Potatoes & Corn Salad

SUITABLE
Quick

PREP TIME
15 mins

COOK TIME
15 mins

SERVES
2

Nutrition (per serving)	Kcal	Fat	Sat Fat	Carb	Sugar	Fibre	Protein	Salt
	479	21g	3g	27g	2g	3g	43g	0.5g

INGREDIENTS

1 ½ cup / 200g baby new potatoes

1 sweetcorn cob

2 skinless salmon fillets

⅓ cup / 60g tomatoes

For the dressing

1 tbsp red wine vinegar

1 tbsp extra-virgin olive oil

1 shallot, finely chopped

1 tbsp capers, finely chopped

handful basil leaves

METHOD

01/ Cook potatoes in boiling water until tender, adding corn for final 5 minutes. Drain & cool.

02/ For the dressing, mix the vinegar, oil, shallot, capers, basil & seasoning.

03/ Heat grill to high. Rub some dressing on salmon & cook, skinned-side down, for 7-8 minutes. Slice tomatoes & place on plate. Slice the potatoes, cut the corn from the cob & add to plate. Add the salmon & drizzle over the remaining dressing.

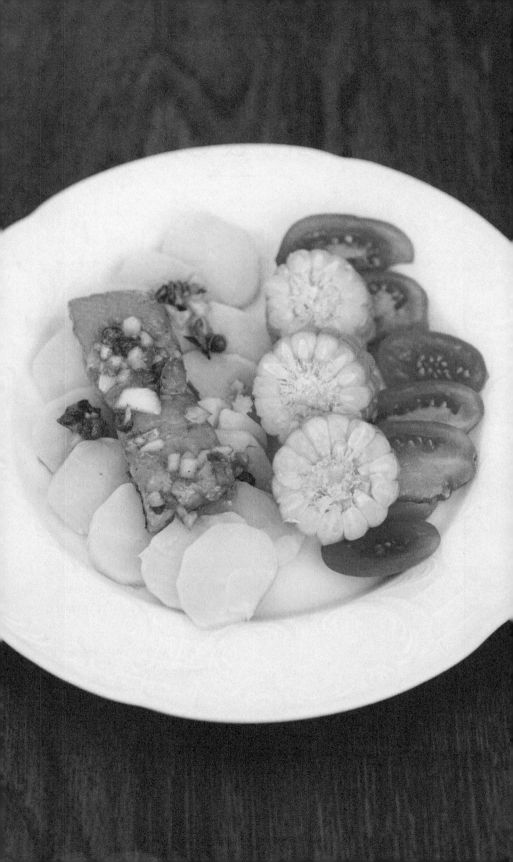

Crusted Cod with Pesto & Olives

SUITABLE	**PREP TIME**	**COOK TIME**	**SERVES**
Quick	5 mins	15 mins	2

Nutrition (per serving)	Kcal	Fat	Sat Fat	Carb	Sugar	Fibre	Protein	Salt
	219	4g	1g	17g	1g	1g	30g	1.1g

INGREDIENTS

1 tbsp green pesto

finely grated zest ½ lemon

5 olives, pitted & chopped

¼ cup / 40g fresh breadcrumbs

2 cod fillets

METHOD

01/ Heat oven to 400F (200C). Mix the pesto, lemon zest & olives together, then stir in the breadcrumbs.

02/ Lay the fish fillets on a baking tray, skinside down, then press the crumbs over the surface of each piece. Bake in the oven for 10-12 minutes until the fish is cooked through and the crust is crisp and brown.

03/ Serve with roasted vegetables and green salad.

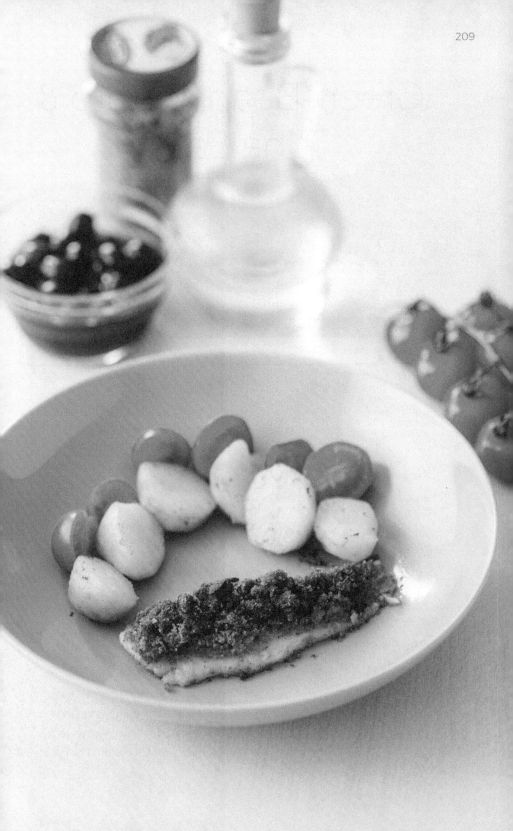

Green Bean, Potato & Tuna Salad

SUITABLE

Quick

PREP TIME

10 mins

COOK TIME

15 mins

SERVES

2

Nutrition (per serving)	Kcal	Fat	Sat Fat	Carb	Sugar	Fibre	Protein	Salt
	284	8g	1g	30g	2g	5g	26g	0.2g

INGREDIENTS

1 cup / 150g new potatoes

1 ½ / 200g green beans, trimmed and halved

5-6 oz / 160g can tuna in water, drained

handful rocket leaves / arugula

For the dressing

1 tsp harissa paste

½ tbsp red wine vinegar

1 tbsp olive oil

METHOD

01 / Put the potatoes in a pan of boiling water, then boil for 6-8 minutes until almost tender. Add beans, then cook for a further 5 minutes until everything is cooked.

02 / Meanwhile, whisk together the harissa and vinegar in a small bowl with seasoning. Add oil until the dressing is thickened. Drain potatoes well, toss with half of the dressing, then leave to cool.

03 / Flake the tuna, then fold into the potatoes. Add the remaining dressing, then gently toss. Divide between 2 bowls and serve each portion with a handful of arugula on top.

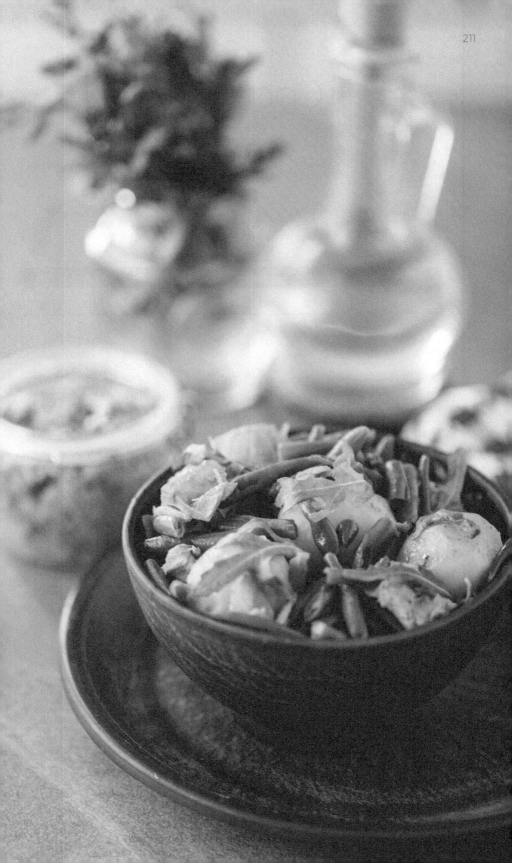

Cod Curry

SUITABLE

Quick

PREP TIME

5 mins

COOK TIME

10 mins

SERVES

2

Nutrition (per serving)	Kcal	Fat	Sat Fat	Carb	Sugar	Fibre	Protein	Salt
	400	14g	2g	38g	10g	5g	33g	1.3g

INGREDIENTS

1 tbsp olive oil

1 onion, chopped

1 garlic clove, chopped

1-2 tbsp Madras curry paste

14 oz / 400g can tomatoes

200ml vegetable stock

2 cod fillets, cut into chunks

1 cup / 200g wholegrain rice

METHOD

01/ Heat the oil in a deep pan and gently fry the onion and garlic for about 5 mins until soft. Add the curry paste and fry for 1-2 minutes, then tip in the tomatoes and stock.

02/ Bring to a simmer, then add the fish. Gently cook for 4-5 minutes until the fish flakes easily. Serve immediately with rice.

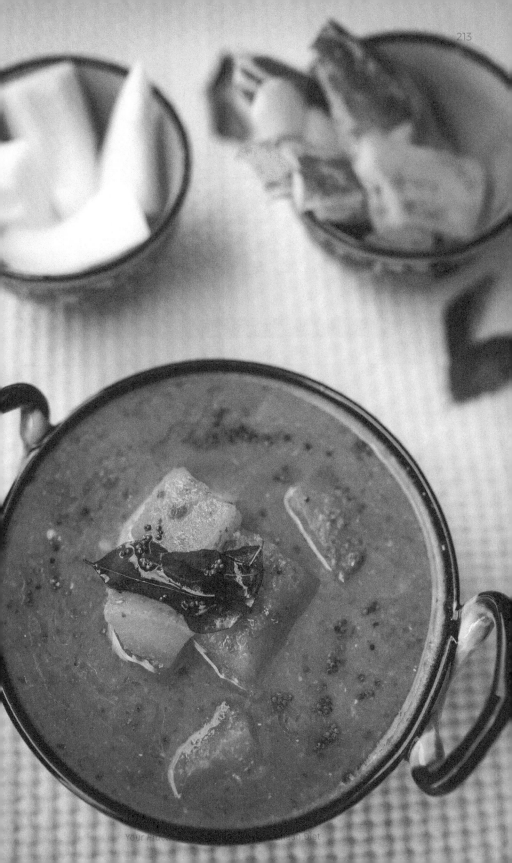

Trout with Couscous & Almonds

SUITABLE

Quick

PREP TIME

10 mins

COOK TIME

20 mins

SERVES

2

Nutrition (per serving)	Kcal	Fat	Sat Fat	Carb	Sugar	Fibre	Protein	Salt
	413	19g	3g	21g	0g	2g	37g	0.2g

INGREDIENTS

⅔ cup / 150ml hot vegetable stock

¼ cup / 50g couscous

1 tbsp almonds

2 tbsp chopped parsley

1 lemon, zest and juice

1 tbsp olive oil, for greasing

4 boneless trout fillets

METHOD

01/ Pour the stock over the couscous in a bowl, cover with cling film and leave until the stock has been absorbed. Add the almonds into the couscous with parsley, lemon zest and juice and season.

02/ Heat oven to 400F (200C). Lightly oil 2 sheets of foil. Season the trout, then make 2 'sandwiches' of 2 fillets with the couscous in the middle. Repeat with the rest of the trout and the couscous. Wrap the 'sandwiches' individually in foil, then bake for 15-20 minutes. Serve with potatoes and salad.

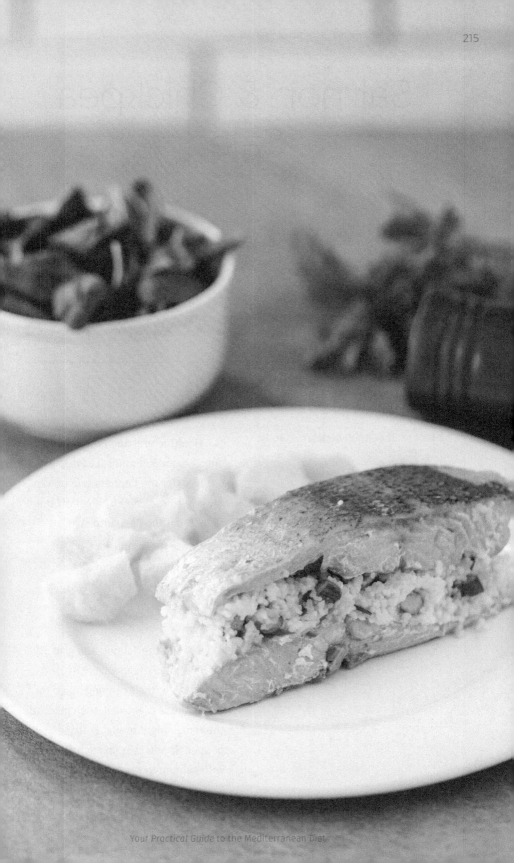

Salmon & Chickpea Salad

SUITABLE
Quick

PREP TIME
5 mins

COOK TIME
15 mins

SERVES
2

Nutrition (per serving)	Kcal	Fat	Sat Fat	Carb	Sugar	Fibre	Protein	Salt
	564	21g	3g	52g	3g	11g	47g	1.8g

INGREDIENTS

1 large red pepper, quartered and deseeded

½ lemon, zest and juice

pinch smoked paprika

1 tbsp extra-virgin olive oil

3 ⅓ cup / 100g baby spinach

2 salmon fillets

14 oz / 400g can chickpeas

METHOD

01 / Heat the grill and grill the pepper quarters for 5 minutes. Leave the grill on. Transfer the peppers to a bowl & leave to cool slightly. Peel off the skins & cut the flesh into strips.

02 / Whisk the lemon zest, juice, smoked paprika, olive oil & seasoning. Toss half the dressing with the spinach leaves and divide between 2 bowls.

03 / Season the salmon and grill for 5 minutes. Meanwhile, heat the chickpeas in their canning liquid for 3-4 minutes, drain well, then mix with the remaining dressing & strips of pepper. Spoon over spinach and top with salmon to serve.

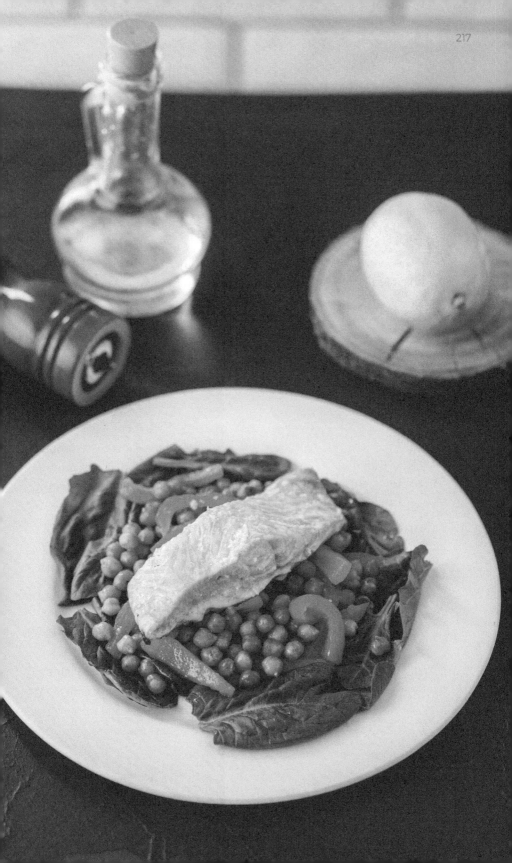

Haddock with Spiced Bulgur Wheat

SUITABLE
High Protein

PREP TIME
10 mins

COOK TIME
35 mins

SERVES
2

Nutrition (per serving)	Kcal	Fat	Sat Fat	Carb	Sugar	Fibre	Protein	Salt
	385	11g	1g	30g	12g	7g	42g	0.8g

INGREDIENTS

1 tbsp olive oil

1 onion, finely sliced

2 carrots, grated

1 tsp cumin seed

1 tbsp harissa

½ cup / 100g bulgur wheat

3 dried apricot, chopped

1 vegetable stock cube

3 ⅓ cup / 100g baby spinach

2 haddock fillets

METHOD

01 / Heat the oil in a casserole dish. Tip in the onions and cook for 10 minutes until golden. Add the carrots & cumin & cook for 2 minutes more. Stir through the harissa, bulgur & apricots, pour over the stock & bring to the boil. Cover and simmer for 7 minutes.

02 / Add the spinach & stir through until just wilted. Arrange the haddock fillets on top & season. Replace the lid and cook for 15-16 minutes, keeping over a low heat until the fish is cooked through and the bulgur is tender. Season & serve.

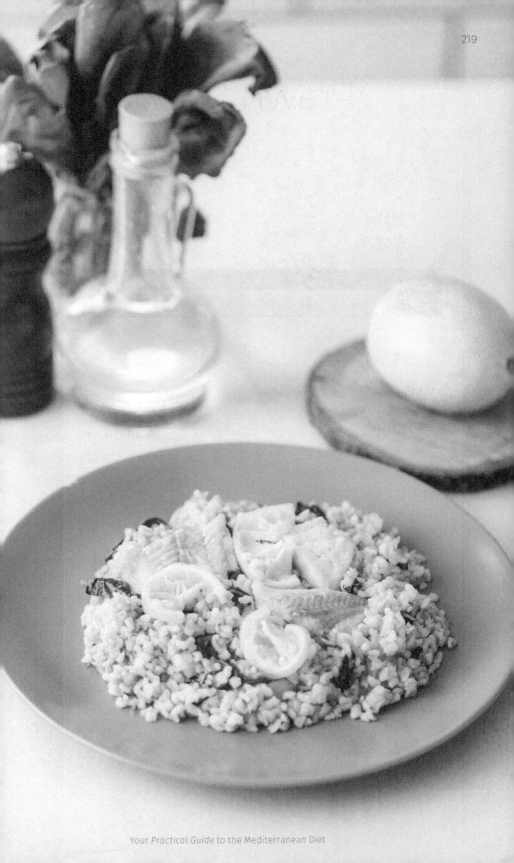

Prawn Stir-Fry

SUITABLE

PREP TIME
10 mins

COOK TIME
40 mins

SERVES
2

Nutrition (per serving)	Kcal	Fat	Sat Fat	Carb	Sugar	Fibre	Protein	Salt
	280	18g	4g	6g	3g	2g	25g	1.8g

INGREDIENTS

1 tbsp oil

3.5 oz / 100g cooked prawns, defrosted if frozen

thumb-sized knob of ginger

large handful fresh beansprouts

4 spring onions, sliced

4 eggs, beaten

1 tbsp soy sauce, plus extra to taste

METHOD

01/ Heat the oil in a frying pan and stir-fry the prawns on a high heat for 30 seconds. Add the ginger, bean sprouts and half of the spring onions and stir-fry for another 30 seconds. Change to low heat and pour in the eggs.

02/ Leave to set for a few seconds, then move the egg around the pan with a spatula to scramble. When the egg sets, add soy sauce. Serve sprinkled with the rest of the sliced spring onion & season with more soy sauce to taste.

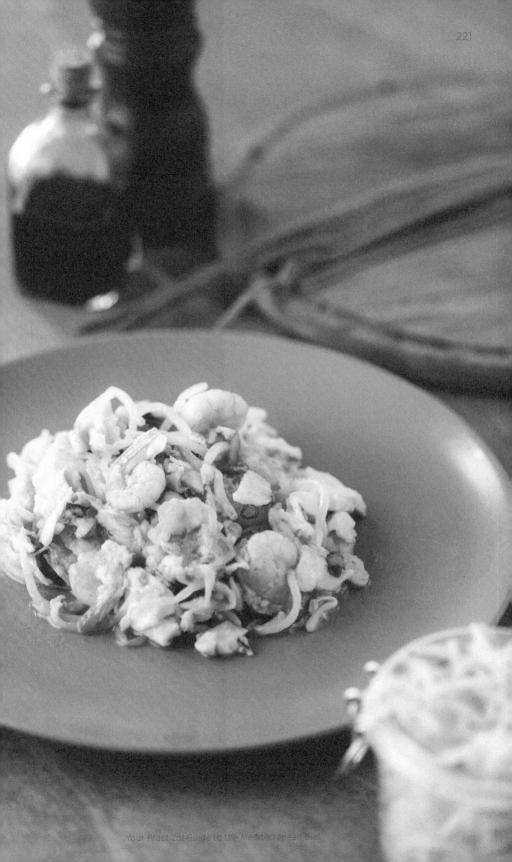

Prawn, Tomato & Pea Spaghetti

SUITABLE
Quick

PREP TIME
5 mins

COOK TIME
15 mins

SERVES
2

Nutrition (per serving)	Kcal	Fat	Sat Fat	Carb	Sugar	Fibre	Protein	Salt
	383	2g	1g	56g	8g	6g	28g	1.6g

INGREDIENTS

3 tbsp frozen peas

1 tsp olive oil

½ onion, diced

1 tsp dried thyme

½ tin of tomatoes

1 tsp salt

7 oz / 200g cooked prawns

1 cup / 200g dried spaghetti

pea shoots, to serve

METHOD

01 / Cook the spaghetti as per the packet instructions.

02 / In a saucepan, heat the oil. Add the onion and stir for 3-4 minutes, until soft. Add the tin tomatoes, thyme and salt and simmer until thickened a little.

03 / Add the peas (no need to defrost) and heat in the sauce until heated through. Add the prawns and heat for 3-4 minutes. Don't leave for too long or the prawns will become tough. Add the cooked spaghetti to the pan and coat in the sauce.

04 / Divide between 2 plates. Serve immediately with pea shoots.

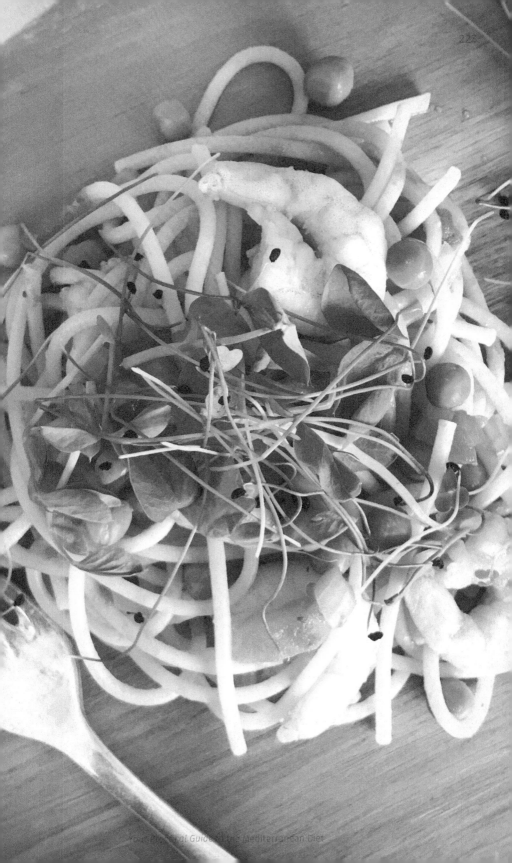

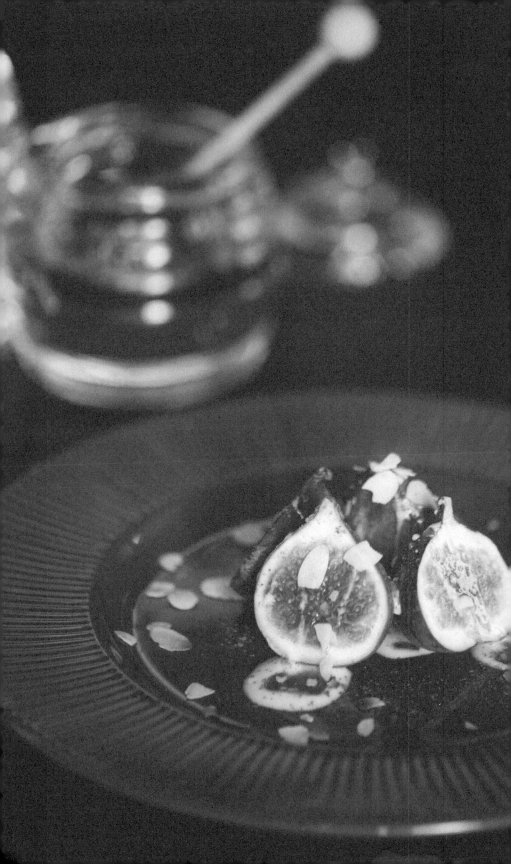

Snacks / Sides

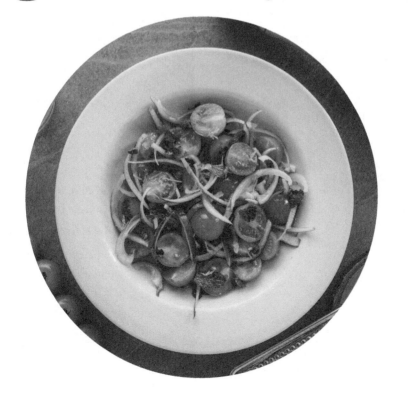

Herbed Baked Potatoes

SUITABLE

Vegetarian

PREP TIME

5 mins

COOK TIME

40 mins

SERVES

2

Nutrition (per serving)	Kcal	Fat	Sat Fat	Carb	Sugar	Fibre	Protein	Salt
	181	7g	1g	28g	1g	3g	4g	1.0g

INGREDIENTS

1 tbsp olive oil

1 tsp salt

2 garlic cloves, bashed, left in skins

1 small bunch of fresh dill, roughly chopped

1 small bunch of fresh parsley, roughly chopped

1 small bunch of fresh chives

2 large floury potatoes, chopped into 1-2cm dice

METHOD

01 / Pre-heat the oven to 400F (200C). Place a baking tray in the oven with the oil and garlic.

02 / After 5 minutes, remove the tin and add the cubed potatoes. Bake for 30 minutes.

03 / Remove from the oven, give a good shake and return for another 5 minutes at 425F (220C). When golden and crisp, remove from the oven. Remove the garlic and stir through the fresh herbs.

04 / Serve immediately, or store in the fridge and crisp up in the oven for 5-10 minutes for up to 5 days later.

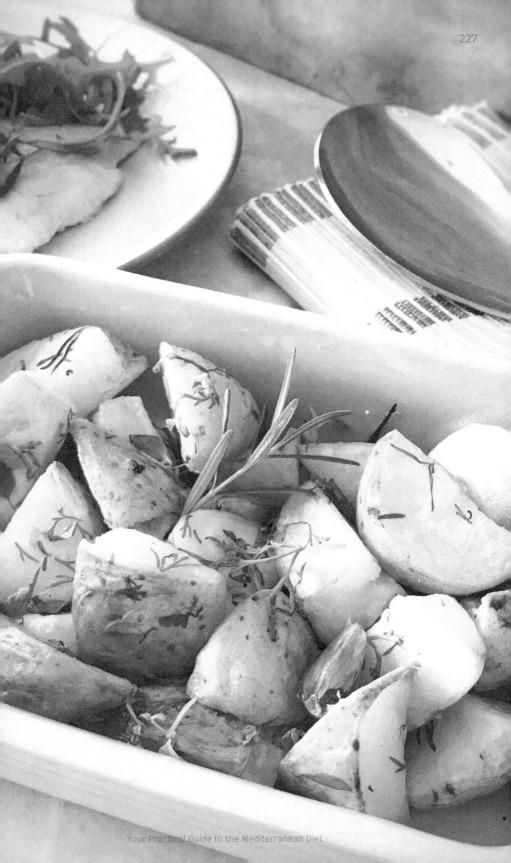

Lemon, Chickpea & Protein Rice

SUITABLE	**PREP TIME**	**COOK TIME**	**SERVES**
Vegetarian	5 mins	10 mins	2

Nutrition (per serving)	Kcal	Fat	Sat Fat	Carb	Sugar	Fibre	Protein	Salt
	300	10g	1g	41g	3g	10g	11g	0.4g

INGREDIENTS

1 ¼ cup / 250g ready cooked puy lentils pouch

1 ¼ cup / 250g ready cooked lemon basmati pouch *(or just a plain one)*

2 tbsp chickpeas

1 tsp olive oil

½ onion, chopped finely

1 lemon, zest only

1 tbsp sunflower seeds

1 tsp chopped fresh mint leaves

METHOD

01/ In a saucepan, heat the oil. Add the onion and stir for 3-4 minutes, until soft. Add all of the other ingredients, except the mint leaves and stir until piping hot. Add a splash of water if the rice begins to stick.

02/ Divide between plates and scatter over the mint leaves.

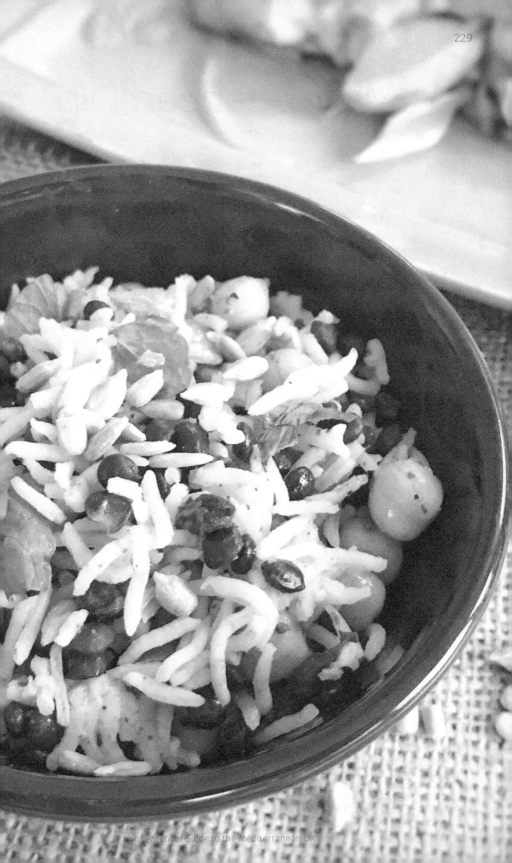

Mediterranean Dip

SUITABLE
Vegetarian

PREP TIME
10 mins

COOK TIME
0 mins

SERVES
4

Nutrition (per serving)	Kcal	Fat	Sat Fat	Carb	Sugar	Fibre	Protein	Salt
	213	12g	7g	16g	2g	4g	12g	1.5g

INGREDIENTS

14 oz / 400g can cannellini bean

1 ⅓ cup / 200g feta cheese

1 tbsp lemon juice

1 garlic clove, crushed

3 tbsp chopped dill, mint or chives
(or 1 tbsp each)

METHOD

01/ Drain and rinse beans. Tip into a food processor with feta, lemon juice and garlic. Whizz until smooth. Add dill, mint or chives, and season with pepper.

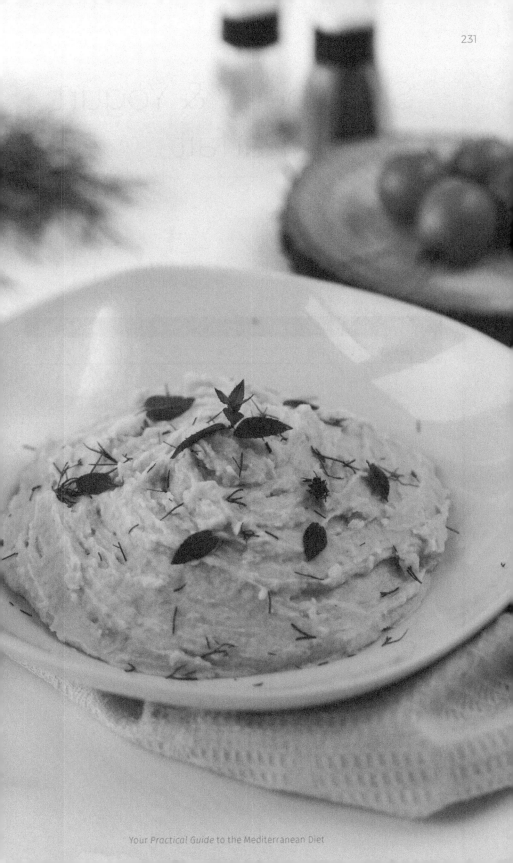

Strawberry & Yogurt Parfait

SUITABLE	**PREP TIME**	**COOK TIME**	**SERVES**
Vegetarian	5 mins	0 mins	2

Nutrition (per serving)	Kcal	Fat	Sat Fat	Carb	Sugar	Fibre	Protein	Salt
	161	4g	1g	23g	13g	2g	9g	0.1g

INGREDIENTS

11 cup / 50g punnet strawberries, chopped

1 tbsp sugar

⅔ cup / 150g Greek yogurt

4 small amaretti biscuit, crushed

METHOD

01/ In a small bowl, mix the strawberries with half the sugar, then roughly mash them with a fork. Mix the remaining sugar into the yogurt, then layer up 6 glasses with amaretti biscuits, yogurt and strawberries.

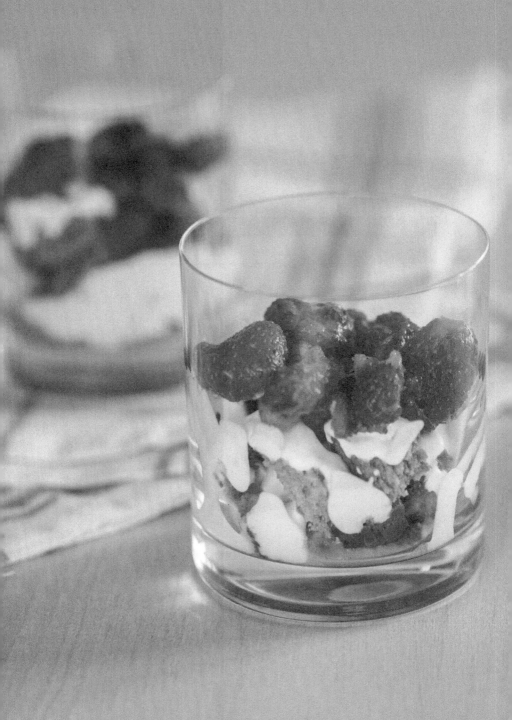

Pea & Artichoke Hummus

SUITABLE
Vegetarian

PREP TIME
10 mins

COOK TIME
0 mins

SERVES
4

Nutrition (per serving)	Kcal	Fat	Sat Fat	Carb	Sugar	Fibre	Protein	Salt
	52	4g	1g	4g	1g	2g	1g	0.1g

INGREDIENTS

½ cup / 70g frozen peas

⅓ cup / 50g artichoke hearts

1 tsp ground cumin

1 tbsp lemon juice

1 tbsp olive oil

small handful mint leaves

METHOD

01/ Tip the peas into a bowl and pour over boiling water to cover. Leave for 5 mins, then drain well and tip into a food processor with all the other ingredients and seasoning. Blend to make a rough purée, then spoon into a small bowl. Cover with cling film, chill until ready to serve.

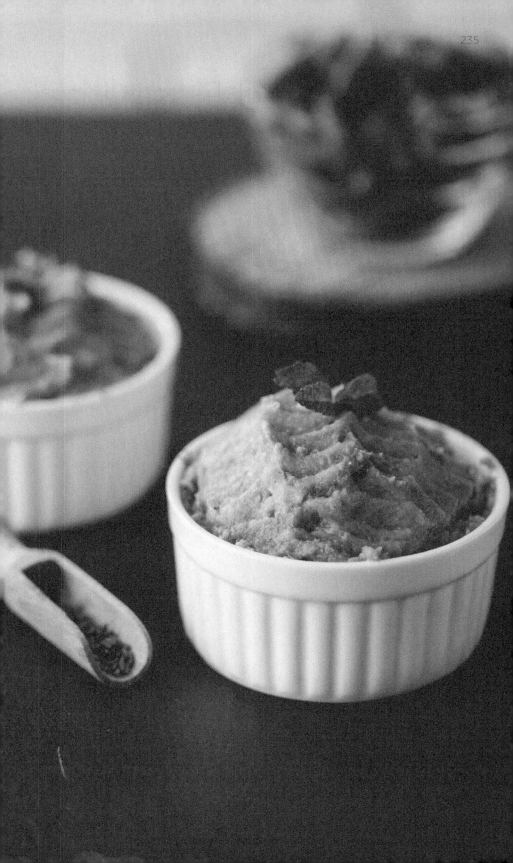

Honeyed Figs with Yogurt & Almonds

SUITABLE

Vegetarian

PREP TIME

5 mins

COOK TIME

0 mins

SERVES

1

Nutrition (per serving)	Kcal	Fat	Sat Fat	Carb	Sugar	Fibre	Protein	Salt
	151	5g	1g	24g	11g	2g	4g	0.1g

INGREDIENTS

2 figs

2 tbsp Greek yogurt

1 tbsp honey

2 pinches of cinnamon

handful flaked toasted almonds

METHOD

01/ Cut the figs in half. Spoon over the yogurt, then drizzle with honey. Sprinkle with cinnamon and a few flaked toasted almonds.

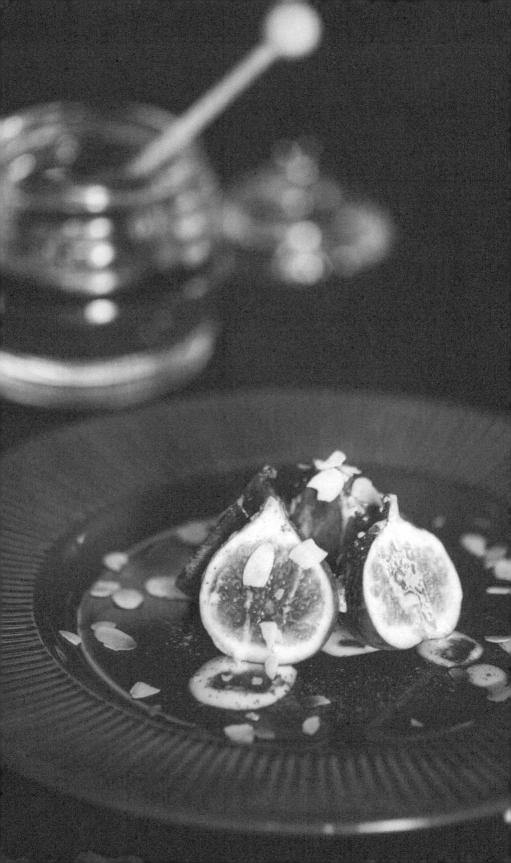

Minty Toms Salad

SUITABLE	**PREP TIME**	**COOK TIME**	**SERVES**
Vegetarian	10 mins	0 mins	3

Nutrition (per serving)	Kcal	Fat	Sat Fat	Carb	Sugar	Fibre	Protein	Salt
	60	5g	1g	4g	2g	1g	1g	0g

INGREDIENTS

1 ⅓ cup / 200g cherry tomatoes

½ red onion

handful of mint leaves

extra-virgin olive oil, for drizzling

lemon zest

METHOD

01/ Halve the tomatoes and scatter over a plate. Finely chop the red onion and tear up the mint leaves. Throw the onion and mint over the tomatoes.

02/ Just before serving, drizzle with extra virgin olive oil, season with salt and ground black pepper and finely grate a little lemon zest over the top.

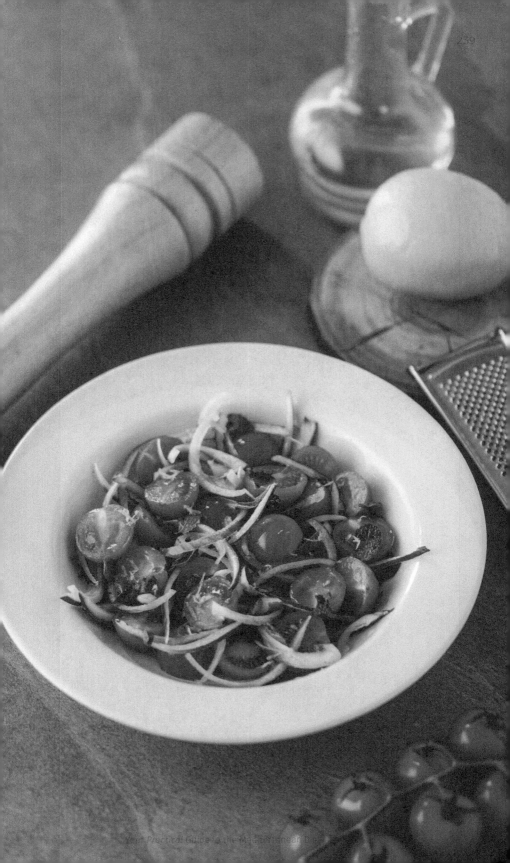

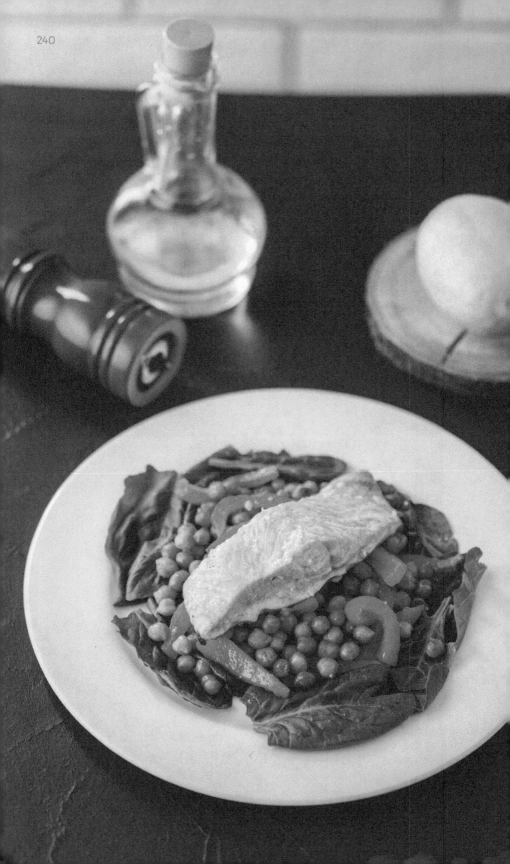

28 Day Plan

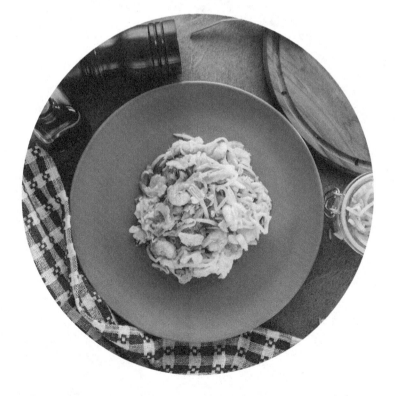

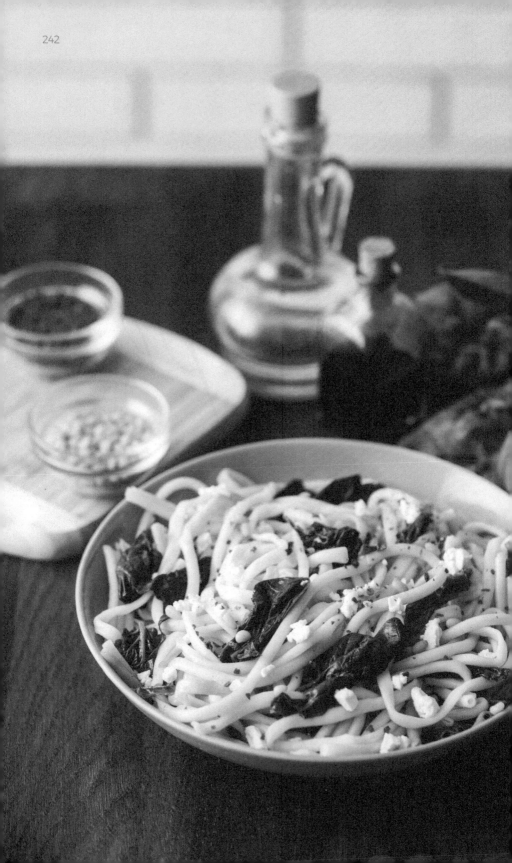

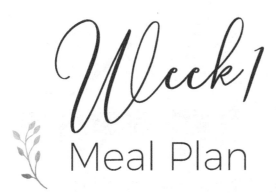

Meal Plan

	BREAKFAST	LUNCH	DINNER
MON	Tomato & Feta Omelette (page 30)	Mixed Bean Salad (62)	Crusted Cod with Pesto & Olives (208)
TUE	Breakfast Blues Porridge (26)	Edgy Veggie Wraps (64)	Pollo Español Hornear (144)
WED	Berry Smoothie (28)	Speedy Couscous Salad (66)	Spinach Spaghetti (94)
THU	Tomato & Feta Omelette (30)	Greek Salad (70)	Green Bean, Potato & Tuna Salad (210)
FRI	Breakfast Blues Porridge (26)	Tangy Couscous Salad (68)	Red Lentil Soup (96)
SAT	Berry Smoothie (28)	Red Lentil Soup (96)	Chicken & Avocado Salad (146)
SUN	Tomato & Feta Omelette (30)	Filler	Grilled Eggplant & Tabbouleh (98)

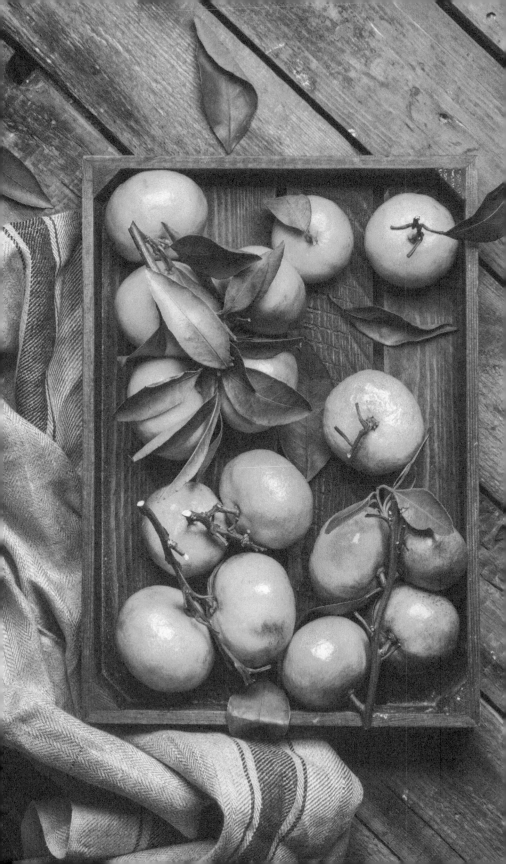

Week 1
Shopping List

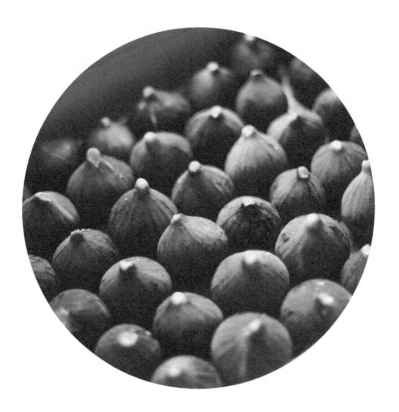

Breakfast & Dinner

This shopping list corresponds to the week 1 meal plan breakfast and dinner recipes, **serving 2 people.**

DAIRY

- [ ] Feta Cheese — 275g / 10 oz
- [ ] Milk — 500 ml / 18 oz
- [ ] Large Eggs — 12
- [ ] Greek Yogurt — 580g / 20 oz

CHILLER

- [ ] Pitted Black Olives — 50g / 2 oz

BAKERY

- [ ] Loaf Granary Bread — 1

MEAT & FISH

- [ ] White Fish (Cod/Hallet) — 2
- [ ] Skinless Chicken Breasts — 4

STORE

- [ ] Whole Wheat Couscous 100g / 3.5 oz
- [ ] Bulgur Wheat — 70g / 2.5 oz
- [ ] Whole Almonds — 100g / 3.5 oz
- [ ] Cumin Seeds
- [ ] Crushed Chilli
- [ ] Vanilla Extract
- [ ] Dried Red Lentils — 140g /5 oz
- [ ] Smoked Paprika
- [ ] Vegetable Stock Cubes — 4
- [ ] Porridge Oats — 125g / 4.5 oz
- [ ] Whole Wheat Spaghetti — 250g / 9 oz

LARDER

- [ ] Honey
- [ ] Can Chickpeas — 400g / 14 oz
- [ ] Red Wine Vinegar
- [ ] Green Pesto
- [ ] Harissa Paste
- [ ] Can Chopped Tomatoes 400g / 14 oz
- [ ] Tuna Chunks in Water — 160g / 5.5 oz
- [ ] Roasted Red Pepper — 10g / 0.5 oz
- [ ] Chia Seeds — 50g / 1.5-2 oz

FRUIT & VEG

- [ ] Red Onions — 4
- [ ] Cloves Garlic — 3
- [ ] Fresh Flat-Leaf Parsley
- [ ] Blueberries — 300g / 10.5 oz
- [ ] Lemons — 2
- [ ] Rocket Leaves / Arugula
- [ ] New Potatoes — 3 (Just buy 1 kg / 35 oz)
- [ ] Fresh Spinach — 250g / 9 oz
- [ ] Cherry Tomatoes — 390g / 14 oz
- [ ] Green Beans — 175g / 6 oz
- [ ] Salad Leaves (optional) — 120g / 4 oz
- [ ] Fresh Cilantro
- [ ] Fresh Mint
- [ ] Avocado — 1
- [ ] Aubergine / Eggplant — 1
- [ ] Red Pepper — 1

FREEZER

- [ ] Frozen Mixed Berries — 450g / 16 oz

Lunch

This shopping list corresponds to the week 1 meal plan lunch recipes, **serving 2 people.**

DAIRY

☐ Feta Cheese   335 g / 12 oz

CHILLER

☐ Hummus   30 g / 1 oz

BAKERY

☐ Wholemeal Tortillas   2

STORE

☐ Whole Wheat Couscous   300 g / 10.5 oz
☐ Dried Oregano
☐ Vegetable Stock Cubes   3
☐ Almonds   20 g / 1 oz

LARDER

☐ Extra-virgin Olive Oil
☐ Can Cannellini Beans   200 g / 7 oz
☐ Sun-Dried Tomato Paste
☐ Red Wine Vinegar
☐ Pesto   30 g / 1 oz
☐ Black Olives   54 g / 2 oz
☐ Artichokes in Oil   140 g / 5 oz

FRUIT & VEG

☐ Red Pepper   1
☐ Red Onion   1
☐ Spring Onions   3
☐ Fresh Flat-Leaf Parsley
☐ Zucchini / Courgettes   2
☐ Cucumbers   3
☐ Lemon   1
☐ Cherry Tomatoes   550 g / 19.5 oz

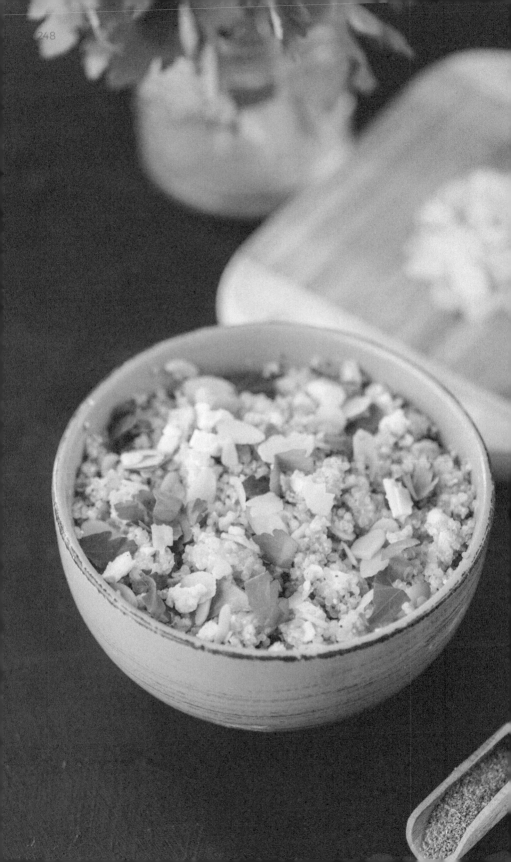

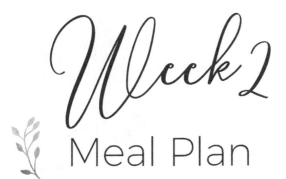

Meal Plan

	BREAKFAST	LUNCH	DINNER
MON	Apple & Blueberry Bircher Pots (page 36)	Mixed Bean Salad (62)	Trout with Couscous & Almonds (214)
TUE	Zucchini, Feta & Mint Salad (34)	Edgy Veggie Wraps (64)	Chicken & Peach Fusion (150)
WED	Sardines on Toast (32)	Speedy Couscous Salad (66)	Bean, Chickpea & Pepper Salad (102)
THU	Apple & Blueberry Bircher Pots (36)	Greek Salad (70)	Citrus Chicken & Couscous (148)
FRI	Zucchini, Feta & Mint Salad (34)	Tangy Couscous Salad (66)	Spicy Quinoa & Almond Salad (104)
SAT	Sardines on Toast (32)	Spicy Quinoa Almond Salad (104)	Greek Salad Omelette (100)
SUN	Apple & Blueberry Bircher Pots (36)	Filler	Chickpea, Pepper & Spiced Bulgar Wheat (106)

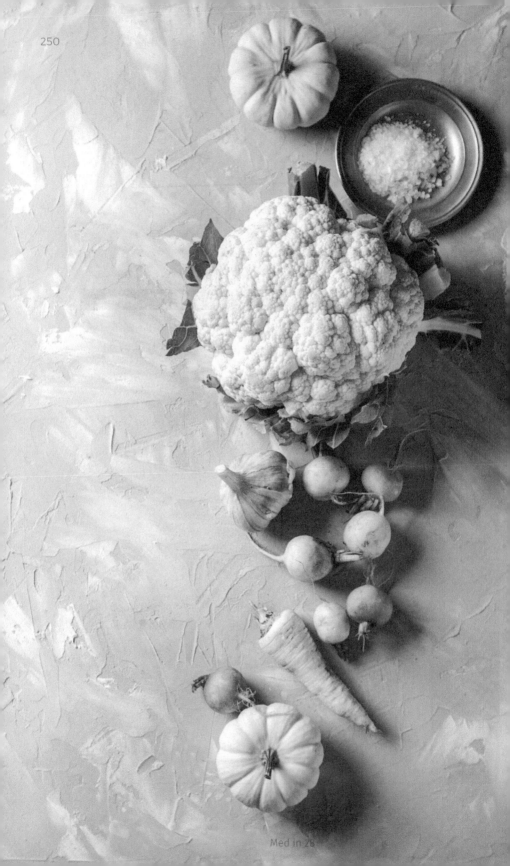

Week 2

Shopping List

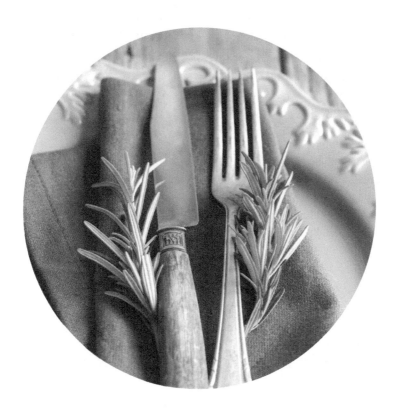

Breakfast & Dinner

This shopping list corresponds to the week 2 meal plan breakfast and dinner recipes, **serving 2 people.**

DAIRY

- [ ] Feta Cheese — 350 g / 12.5 oz
- [ ] Eggs — 5
- [ ] Greek Yogurt — 180 g / 6.5 oz

BAKERY

- [ ] Brown Bread — 360 g / 12.5 oz

MEAT & FISH

- [ ] Chicken Breast — 500 g / 17.5 oz
- [ ] Trout Fillets — 440 g / 15.5 oz

STORE

- [ ] Bulgur Wheat — 300 g / 10.5 oz
- [ ] Whole Wheat Couscous — 300 g / 10.5 oz
- [ ] Flaked Almonds — 60 g / 2 oz
- [ ] Oats — 65 g / 2.5 oz
- [ ] Ras el Hanout
- [ ] Crushed Chilli
- [ ] Vegetable Stock Cubes — 3
- [ ] Ground Cilantro
- [ ] Ground Turmeric
- [ ] Ground Cumin
- [ ] Ground Cinnamon
- [ ] Quinoa — 150 g / 5 oz

LARDER

- [ ] Sardines — 480 g / 17 oz
- [ ] Extra-virgin Olive Oil
- [ ] Can Chickpeas — 1000 g / 35 oz
- [ ] Red Wine Vinegar

- [ ] Sultanas — 42 g / 1.5 oz
- [ ] Green Pesto — 15 g / 0.5 oz
- [ ] Black Olives — 55 g / 2 oz
- [ ] Honey
- [ ] Roasted Red Peppers — 220 g / 7.5 oz

FRUIT & VEG

- [ ] Red Onions — 1
- [ ] Cloves Garlic — 4
- [ ] Fresh Red Chillies — 3
- [ ] Fresh Flat-Leaf Parsley — 32 g ./ 1 oz
- [ ] Apples — 6
- [ ] Blueberries — 120 g / 4 oz
- [ ] Courgettes — 2
- [ ] Lemons — 6
- [ ] Rocket Leaves / Arugula — 100 g / 3.5 oz
- [ ] Peaches — 2
- [ ] Cherry Tomatoes — 200 g / 7 oz
- [ ] Green Beans — 200 g / 7 oz
- [ ] Fresh Mint — 25 g / 1 oz
- [ ] Herb Salad — 55 g / 2 oz

Lunch

This shopping list corresponds to the week 2 meal plan lunch recipes, **serving 2 people.**

DAIRY

☐ Feta Cheese   335 g /12 oz

CHILLER

☐ Hummus   30 g / 1 oz

BAKERY

☐ Wholemeal Tortillas   2

STORE

☐ Whole Wheat Couscous   300 g / 10.5 oz
☐ Dried Oregano
☐ Vegetable Stock Cubes   3
☐ Almonds   20 g / 1 oz

LARDER

☐ Extra-virgin Olive Oil
☐ Can Cannellini Beans   200 g / 7 oz
☐ Sun-Dried Tomato Paste
☐ Red Wine Vinegar
☐ Pesto   30 g /1 oz
☐ Black Olives   54 g /2 oz
☐ Artichokes in Oil   140 g / 5 oz

FRUIT & VEG

☐ Red Pepper   1
☐ Red Onion   1
☐ Spring Onions   3
☐ Fresh Flat-Leaf Parsley
☐ Zucchinis / Courgettes   2
☐ Cucumbers   3
☐ Lemon   1
☐ Cherry Tomatoes   550 g / 19.5 oz

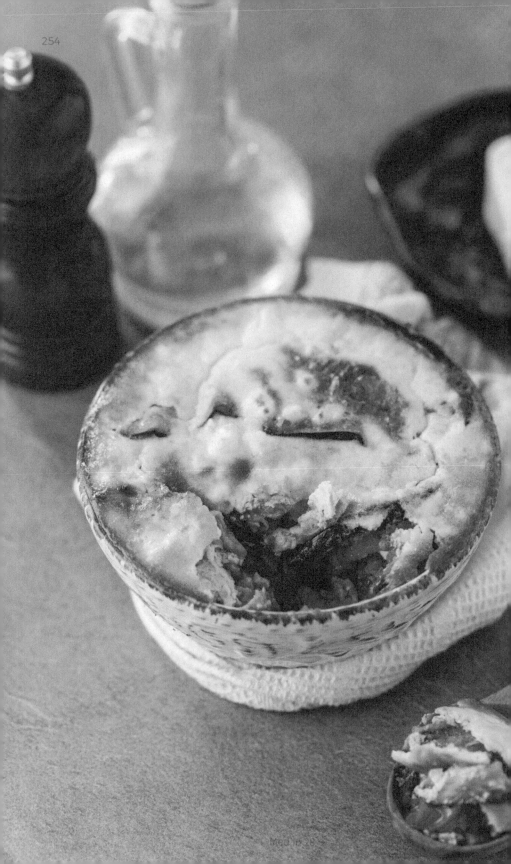

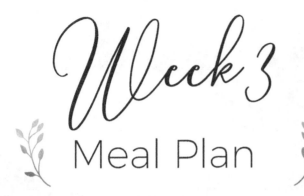

Week 3
Meal Plan

	BREAKFAST	LUNCH	DINNER
MON	Basil & Spinach Scramble (page 42)	Mixed Bean Salad (62)	Salmon & Chikpea Salad (216)
TUE	Banana Yogurt Pots (40)	Edgy Veggie Wraps (64)	Roast Carrot & Bean Salad with Feta (108)
WED	Blueberry Oats Bowl (38)	Speedy Couscous Salad (66)	Moussaka (174)
THU	Basil & Spinach Scramble (42)	Greek Salad (70)	Chicken & Ham with New Potatoes (156)
FRI	Banana Yogurt Pots (40)	Tangy Couscous Salad (68)	Stuffed Peppers (116)
SAT	Blueberry Oats Bowl (38)	Stuffed Peppers	Grilled Eggplant Slices with Hummus (114)
SUN	Basil & Spinach Scramble (42)	Filler	Patatas Bravas with Chorizo (194)

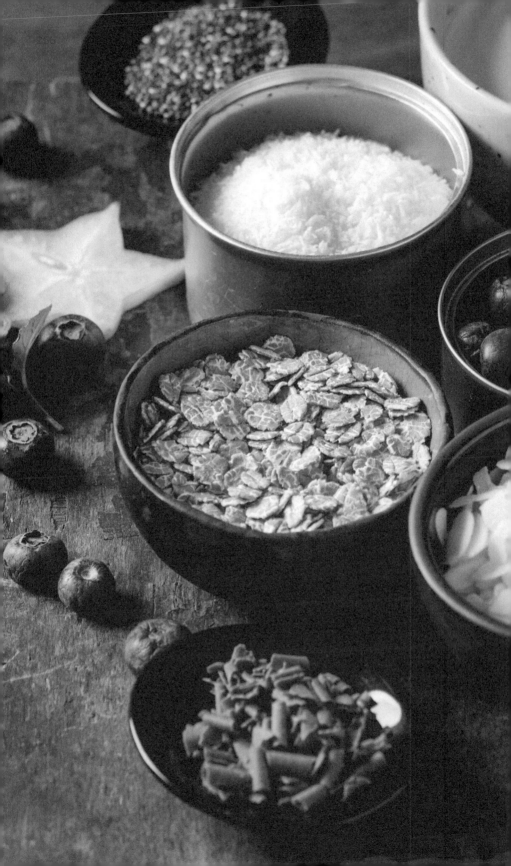

Week 3

Shopping List

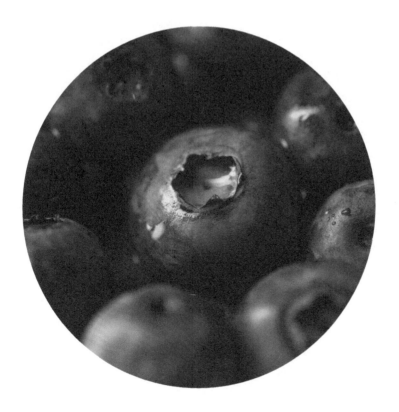

Breakfast & Dinner

This shopping list corresponds to the week 3 meal plan breakfast and dinner recipes, **serving 2 people.**

DAIRY

☐ Feta Cheese	200 g / 7 oz
☐ Large Eggs	13
☐ Fat Free Greek Yogurt	1000 g / 35 oz

CHILLER

☐ Prosciutto	25 g /1 oz
☐ Hummus	150 g / 5 oz
☐ Cooking Chorizo	125 g / 4.5 oz

BAKERY

☐ Wholemeal Loaf	

MEAT & FISH

☐ Chicken Breasts	2
☐ Lean Beef Mince	250 g / 9 oz
☐ Salmon Fillets	2

STORE

☐ Pepper	
☐ Walnuts	125 g / 4.5 oz
☐ Couscous	140 g / 5 oz
☐ Porridge Oats	70 g / 2.5 oz
☐ Paprika	

LARDER

☐ Honey	
☐ Can Butter Beans	200 g /7 oz
☐ Tinned Chopped Tomatoes	400 g / 14 oz
☐ Extra-virgin Olive Oil	
☐ Can Chickpeas	400 g / 14 oz
☐ Sun-Dried Tomato Paste	
☐ Black Olives	40 g / 1.5 oz

FRUIT & VEG

☐ Red Peppers	5
☐ Red Onion	2
☐ Cloves Garlic	2
☐ Fresh Red Chillies	1
☐ Fresh Basil	35 g /1 oz
☐ Fresh Flat-Leaf Parsley	20 g / 0.5 oz
☐ Aubergines / Eggplant	2
☐ Bananas	4
☐ New Potatoes	1 kg / 35 oz
☐ Fresh Mint	10 g / 0.5 oz
☐ Cherry Tomatoes	800 g / 28 oz
☐ Green Beans	200 g / 7 oz
☐ Baby Spinach	600 g / 21 oz
☐ Baby Carrots	500 g / 17.5 oz
☐ Lemons	2

FREEZER

☐ Frozen Blueberries	350 g / 12 oz

Lunch

This shopping list corresponds to the week 3 meal plan lunch recipes, **serving 2 people.**

DAIRY

☐ Feta Cheese   335 g / 12 oz

CHILLER

☐ Hummus   30 g / 1 oz

BAKERY

☐ Wholemeal Tortillas   2

STORE

☐ Whole Wheat Couscous   300 g / 10.5 oz

☐ Dried Oregano

☐ Vegetable Stock Cubes   3

☐ Almonds   20 g / 1 oz

LARDER

☐ Extra-virgin Olive Oil

☐ Tinned Cannellini Beans   200 g / 7 oz

☐ Sun-Dried Tomato Paste

☐ Red Wine Vinegar

☐ Pesto   30 g / 1 oz

☐ Black Olives   54 g / 2 oz

☐ Artichokes in Oil   140 g / 5 oz

FRUIT & VEG

☐ Red Pepper   1

☐ Red Onion   1

☐ Spring Onions   3

☐ Fresh Flat-Leaf Parsley

☐ Zucchinis / Courgettes   2

☐ Cucumbers   3

☐ Lemon   1

☐ Cherry Tomatoes   550 g / 19.5 oz

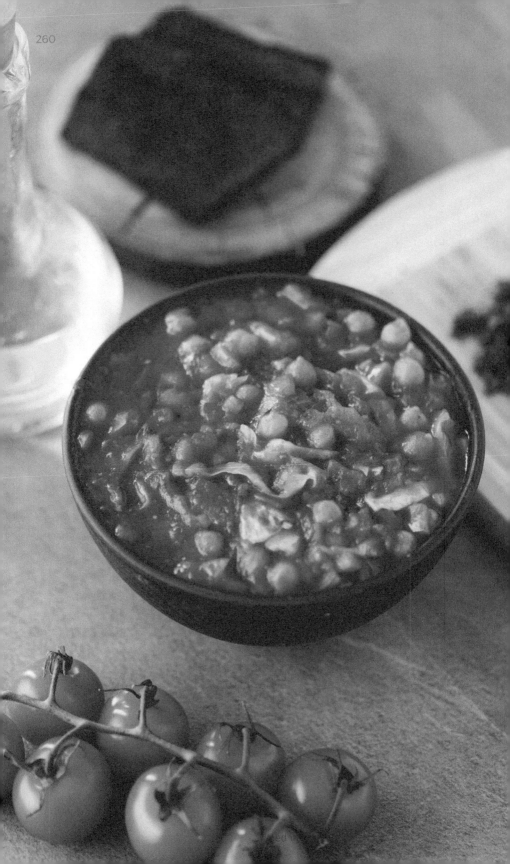

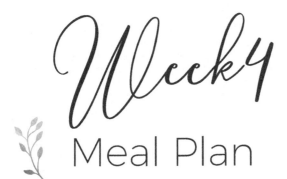

Meal Plan

	BREAKFAST	LUNCH	DINNER
MON	Fruity Bircher Muesli (page 44)	Mixed Bean Salad (62)	Morrocan Chicken & Sweet Potato Mash (158)
TUE	Veggie Stir Fry Omelette (48)	Edgy Veggie Wraps (64)	Haddock with Spiced Bulgur Wheat (218)
WED	Strawberry & Almond Smoothie (46)	Speedy Couscous Salad (66)	Squash & Lentil Salad (122)
THU	Fruity Bircher Muesli (44)	Traditional Greek Salad (70)	Eggplant Lentil Bake (118)
FRI	Veggie Stir Fry Omelette (48)	Tangy Couscous Salad (68)	Greek Pasta Salad (124)
SAT	Strawberry & Almond Smoothie (46)	Greek Pasta Salad (124)	Spanish Chorizo & Chickpea Soup (172)
SUN	Fruity Bircher Muesli (44)	Filler	Spicy Tomato Baked Eggs (128)

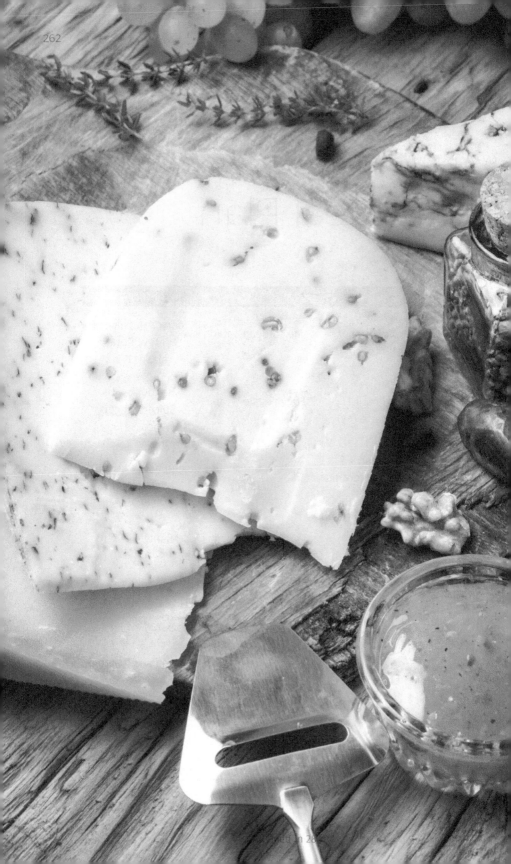

Week 4
Shopping List

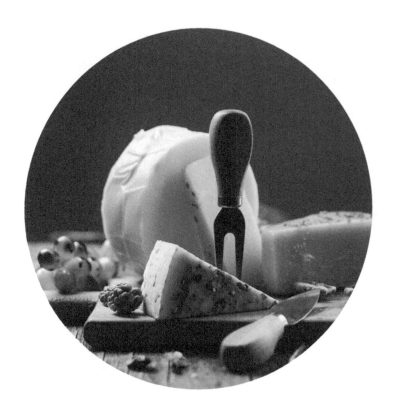

Breakfast & Dinner

This shopping list corresponds to the week 4 meal plan breakfast and dinner recipes, **serving 2 people.**

DAIRY

- [ ] Feta Cheese   240 g / 8.5 oz
- [ ] Milk   200 ml / 8.5 oz oz
- [ ] Eggs   12
- [ ] Greek Yogurt   840 g / 30 oz

CHILLER

- [ ] Chorizo   110 g / 4 oz

MEAT & FISH

- [ ] Chicken Breasts   2
- [ ] Haddock Fillets   280 g / 10 oz

LARDER

- [ ] Extra-virgin Olive Oil
- [ ] Can Chickpeas   410 g / 14 oz
- [ ] Reduced Salt Soy Sauce   60 ml / 2 oz
- [ ] Dried Apricots   12 g / 0.5 oz
- [ ] Lentils   70 g / 2.5 oz
- [ ] Red Wine Vinegar
- [ ] Harissa Paste
- [ ] Black Olives   130 g / 4.5 oz
- [ ] Can Chopped Tomatoes   1400 g / 50 oz
- [ ] Wholegrain Mustard
- [ ] Honey
- [ ] Sultanas   150 g / 5 oz
- [ ] Mixed Seeds   160 g / 5.5 oz
- [ ] Can Lentils   200 g / 7 oz

STORE

- [ ] Bulgur Wheat   100 g / 3.5 oz
- [ ] Ground Cinnamon
- [ ] Ground Almonds   50 g / 2 oz
- [ ] Whole Wheat Fusilli Pasta   300 g / 10.5 oz
- [ ] Ground Cumin
- [ ] Chili Flakes
- [ ] Crushed Chilli
- [ ] Vegetable Stock Cubes   3
- [ ] Cumin Seeds
- [ ] Oats   300 g / 10.5 oz
- [ ] Granary loaf

FRUIT & VEG

- [ ] Red Onions   5
- [ ] Aubergine / Eggplant   1
- [ ] Cloves Garlic   4
- [ ] Fresh Red Chilli   1
- [ ] Apples   6
- [ ] Bananas   10
- [ ] Savoy Cabbage   1
- [ ] Lemon   1
- [ ] Sweet Potatoes   2-4
- [ ] Cherry Tomatoes   325 g / 11.5 oz
- [ ] Fresh Basil   15 g / 0.5 oz
- [ ] Fresh Cilantro   20 g / 0.5 oz
- [ ] Carrots   2-3
- [ ] Butternut Squash   1
- [ ] Strawberries   335 g / 12 oz
- [ ] Baby Spinach   375 g / 13 oz
- [ ] Stir-Fry Vegetables   320 g / 11 oz

$\mathcal{L}$unch

This shopping list corresponds to the week 4 meal plan lunch recipes, **serving 2 people.**

DAIRY

☐ Feta Cheese   335 g / 12 oz

CHILLER

☐ Hummus   30 g / 1 oz

BAKERY

☐ Wholemeal Tortillas   2

STORE

☐ Whole Wheat Couscous   300 g / 10.5 oz
☐ Dried Oregano
☐ Vegetable Stock Cubes   3
☐ Almonds   20 g / 1 oz

LARDER

☐ Extra-virgin Olive Oil
☐ Can Cannellini Beans   200 g / 7 oz
☐ Sun-Dried Tomato Paste
☐ Red Wine Vinegar
☐ Pesto   30 g / 1 oz
☐ Black Olives   54 g / 2 oz
☐ Artichokes in Oil   140 g / 5 oz

FRUIT & VEG

☐ Red Pepper   1
☐ Red Onion   1
☐ Spring Onions   3
☐ Fresh Flat-Leaf Parsley
☐ Zucchinis / Courgettes   2
☐ Cucumbers   3
☐ Lemon   1
☐ Cherry Tomatoes   550 g / 19.5 oz

Good Luck!

———

Thank you for reading my book. I hope that the information provided has helped you further your understanding of the Mediterranean diet.

To learn more recipes and evidence-driven articles on the Mediterranean diet, find us at https://medmunch.com.

To your success,

Alex.

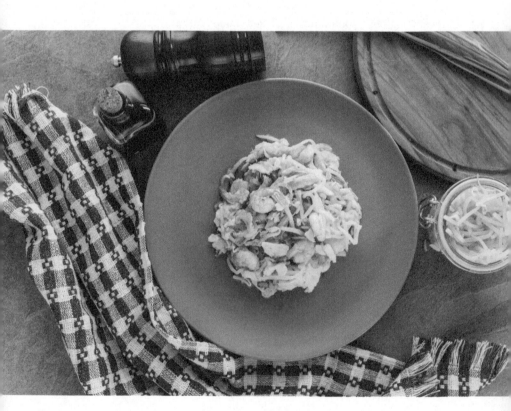

Made in the USA
Coppell, TX
05 July 2023